Contents

COUSCOUS AND CUCUMBER SALAD

Servings: 8 | Prep: 10m | Cooks: 10m | Total: 1h20m

NUTRITION FACTS

Calories: 142 | Carbohydrates: 24.6g | Fat: 3.6g | Protein: 4g | Cholesterol: 0mg

INGREDIENTS

- 10 ounces uncooked couscous
- 1/2 cup finely chopped green onions
- 2 tablespoons olive oil
- 1/2 cup fresh parsley, chopped
- 1/2 cup lemon juice
- 1/4 cup fresh basil, chopped
- 3/4 teaspoon salt
- 6 leaves lettuce
- 1/4 teaspoon ground black pepper
- 6 slices lemon
- 1 cucumber, seeded and chopped
- 1/2 teaspoon lemon pepper

DIRECTIONS

1. In a medium saucepan, bring 1 3/4 cup water to a boil. Stir in couscous; cover. Remove from heat; let stand, covered, 5 minutes. Cool to room temperature.
2. Meanwhile, in a medium bowl combine oil, lemon juice, salt and pepper. Stir in cucumber, green onion, parsley, basil and couscous. Mix well and chill for at least 1 hour.
3. Line a plate with lettuce leaves. Spoon couscous mixture over leaves and garnish with lemon wedges.

HARVESTED CHICKEN STEW

Servings: 10 | Prep: 15m | Cooks: 30m | Total: 45m

NUTRITION FACTS

Calories: 111 | Carbohydrates: 13.1g | Fat: 2.5g | Protein: 10.1g | Cholesterol: 21mg

INGREDIENTS

- 2 cups chopped onion
- 5 cups chicken broth
- 2 cups cubed, cooked boneless chicken breast meat
- 1 cup sweet corn
- 1 cup chopped celery

- 1 cup peas
- 2 cups whole peeled tomatoes, with liquid
- 1 cup sliced zucchini
- 2 cups sliced carrots
- 1/2 teaspoon lemon pepper

DIRECTIONS

1. In a large soup pot combine the onion, chicken, celery, tomatoes with liquid, carrots, broth, corn, peas and zucchini. Stir together and simmer over medium low heat for 1/2 hour, or until vegetables are cooked and tender.

ZESTY ZUCCHINI AND SQUASH
Servings: 6 | Prep: 15m | Cooks: 25m | Total: 40m

NUTRITION FACTS

Calories: 43 | Carbohydrates: 9.7g | Fat: 0.4g | Protein: 1.8g | Cholesterol: 0mg

INGREDIENTS

- 3 medium small yellow squash, cubed
- 1/2 onion, chopped
- 3 small zucchini, cubed
- salt to taste
- 1 (10 ounce) can diced tomatoes with green chile peppers
- garlic powder to taste

DIRECTIONS

1. In a large saucepan, combine squash, zucchini, tomatoes with chiles, onion, salt and garlic powder. Bring to a boil over medium-high heat.
2. Reduce heat to low and cook until tender-crisp.

BANANA OAT BARS
Servings: 18 | Prep: 5m | Cooks: 35m | Total: 45m | Additional: 5m

NUTRITION FACTS

Calories: 72 | Carbohydrates: 16.1g | Fat: 0.5g | Protein: 1.6g | Cholesterol: 0mg

INGREDIENTS

- 1 1/3 cups quick cooking oats
- 1/2 cup raisins

- 1/2 cup white sugar
- 1 cup mashed bananas
- 2 teaspoons baking powder
- 1/4 cup skim milk
- 1 teaspoon ground cinnamon
- 2 egg whites
- 1/2 teaspoon baking soda
- 1 teaspoon vanilla extract

DIRECTIONS

1. Preheat oven to 350 degrees F (175 degrees C).
2. Mix together dry ingredients. In a separate bowl mix together bananas, egg whites, milk and vanilla. Beat all together.
3. Bake in a 9 x 13 inch pan which has been sprayed with non-stick spray for about 35 minutes. Cool and cut into bars. You may sprinkle with cinnamon and sugar, if desired.

GRILLED CORN SALAD

Servings: 6 | Prep: 15m | Cooks: 10m | Total: 1h10m

NUTRITION FACTS

Calories: 103 | Carbohydrates: 19.7g | Fat: 2.8g | Protein: 3.4g | Cholesterol: 0mg

INGREDIENTS

- 6 ears freshly shucked corn
- 1/2 bunch fresh cilantro, chopped, or more to taste
- 1 green pepper, diced
- 2 teaspoons olive oil, or to taste
- 2 Roma (plum) tomatoes, diced
- salt and ground black pepper to taste
- 1/4 cup diced red onion
- 1/2 teaspoon lemon pepper

DIRECTIONS

1. Preheat an outdoor grill for medium heat; lightly oil the grate.
2. Cook the corn on the preheated grill, turning occasionally, until the corn is tender and specks of black appear, about 10 minutes; set aside until just cool enough to handle. Slice the kernels off of the cob and place into a bowl.
3. Combine the warm corn kernels with the green pepper, diced tomato, onion, cilantro, and olive oil. Season with salt and pepper; toss until evenly mixed. Set aside for at least 30 minutes to allow flavors to blend before serving.

MOJITO FRUIT SALAD

Servings: 6 | Prep: 20m | Cooks: 1h | Total: 1h20m

NUTRITION FACTS

Calories: 83 | Carbohydrates: 20.7g | Fat: 0.6g | Protein: 1.3g | Cholesterol: 0mg

INGREDIENTS

- 1 cup cubed seeded watermelon
- 1 cup fresh blueberries
- 1 cup seedless grapes
- 3 sprigs fresh mint
- 1 cup cubed cantaloupe
- 2 teaspoons white sugar
- 1 cup hulled and quartered strawberries
- 3 tablespoons fresh lime juice
- 1 cup peeled and quartered kiwi

DIRECTIONS

1. Mix the watermelon, grapes, cantaloupe, strawberries, and kiwi in a bowl with a tight-fitting lid; top with the blueberries.
2. Stir the mint, sugar, and lime juice together in a bowl, crushing the mint with the back of a spoon while mixing to extract flavors; pour over the fruit mixture. Seal the bowl with lid and refrigerate at least 1 hour.
3. Just before serving, gently flip the sealed bowl several times to coat the fruit with the dressing.

VEGETARIAN BEAN CURRY

Servings: 8 | Prep: 15m | Cooks: 1h10m | Total: 1h25m

NUTRITION FACTS

Calories: 208 | Carbohydrates: 35.9g | Fat: 4.7g | Protein: 8.7g | Cholesterol: 0mg

INGREDIENTS

- 2 tablespoons olive oil
- 1 pinch cayenne pepper
- 1 large white onion, chopped
- 1 (28 ounce) can crushed tomatoes
- 1/2 cup dry lentils
- 1 (15 ounce) can garbanzo beans, drained and rinsed
- 2 cloves garlic, minced
- 1 (8 ounce) can kidney beans, drained and rinsed

- 3 tablespoons curry powder
- 1/2 cup raisins
- 1 teaspoon ground cumin
- salt and pepper to taste

DIRECTIONS

1. Heat the oil in a large pot over medium heat, and cook the onion until tender. Mix in the lentils and garlic, and season with curry powder, cumin, and cayenne pepper. Cook and stir 2 minutes. Stir in the tomatoes, garbanzo beans, kidney beans, and raisins. Season with salt and pepper. Reduce heat to low, and simmer at least 1 hour, stirring occasionally.

PUERTO RICAN TOSTONES
Servings: 2 | Prep: 10m | Cooks: 10m | Total: 20m

NUTRITION FACTS

Calories: 136 | Carbohydrates: 28.5g | Fat: 3.3g | Protein: 1.2g | Cholesterol: 0mg

INGREDIENTS

- 5 tablespoons oil for frying
- 3 cups cold water
- 1 green plantain
- salt to taste

DIRECTIONS

1. Peel the plantain and cut it into 1-inch chunks.
2. Heat the oil in a large skillet. Place the plantains in the oil and fry on both sides,; approximately 3 1/2 minutes per side.
3. Remove the plantains from the pan and flatten the plantains by placing a plate over the fried plantains and pressing down.
4. Dip the plantains in water, then return them to the hot oil and fry 1 minute on each side. Salt to taste and serve immediately.

NO BAKE BUMPY PEANUT BUTTER NUGGETS
Servings: 30 | Prep: 15m | Cooks: 1h | Total: 1h15m

NUTRITION FACTS

Calories: 46 | Carbohydrates: 3.8g | Fat: 2.9g | Protein: 1.9g | Cholesterol: 0mg

INGREDIENTS

- 1/2 cup natural peanut butter
- 1/2 teaspoon ground cinnamon
- 1/4 cup nonfat dry milk powder
- 1/4 cup wheat germ
- 1/4 cup unsweetened flaked coconut
- 1/4 cup unsweetened apple juice concentrate, thawed
- 1/3 cup rolled oats

DIRECTIONS

1. Combine peanut butter, milk powder, and coconut in a large mixing bowl. Stir in oats, ground cinnamon, wheat germ, and apple juice concentrate until thoroughly combined.
2. Shape the mixture into 1 inch balls. Chill thoroughly before serving; store remaining nuggets in the refrigerator.

BAKED BEANS FROM SCRATCH

Servings: 10 | Prep: 10m | Cooks: 8h | Total: 15h30m

NUTRITION FACTS

Calories: 122 | Carbohydrates: 25.9g | Fat: 0.4g | Protein: 4.8g | Cholesterol: 0mg

INGREDIENTS

- 1 cup dried navy beans
- 1 teaspoon Worcestershire sauce
- 4 cups water
- 1/2 teaspoon salt
- 1/4 cup ketchup
- 1/8 teaspoon ground black pepper
- 1/4 cup maple syrup
- 1/8 teaspoon chili powder
- 2 tablespoons brown sugar
- 1 small onion, chopped
- 2 tablespoons molasses

DIRECTIONS

1. Place the navy beans into a large container and cover with several inches of cool water; let stand 8 hours to overnight. Or, bring the beans and water to a boil in a large pot over high heat. Once boiling, turn off the heat, cover, and let stand 1 hour. Drain and rinse before using.
2. Place the beans in a large saucepan with 4 cups of water. Bring to a boil over high heat, then reduce heat to medium-low, cover, and simmer 1 hour.
3. Preheat an oven to 375 degrees F (190 degrees C). Stir the ketchup, maple syrup, brown sugar, molasses, Worcestershire sauce, salt, pepper, and chili powder together in a small bowl; set aside.

4. Once the beans have simmered for 1 hour, drain, and reserve the cooking liquid. Pour the beans into a 1 1/2 quart casserole dish and stir in the chopped onion and the molasses sauce. Stir in enough of the reserved cooking liquid so the sauce covers the beans by 1/4 inch.
5. Cover, and bake in the preheated oven for 10 minutes, then reduce the heat to 200 degrees F (95 degrees C), and cook 6 hours longer. Stir the beans after they have cooked for 3 hours. Once the beans are tender and the sauce has reduced and is sticky, remove from the oven, stir, recover, and allow to stand 15 minutes before serving.

QUINOA CHARD PILAF

Servings: 8 | Prep: 20m | Cooks: 20m | Total: 40m

NUTRITION FACTS

Calories: 224 | Carbohydrates: 36.6g | Fat: 4.7g | Protein: 9.6g | Cholesterol: 0mg

INGREDIENTS

- 1 tablespoon olive oil
- 1 cup canned lentils, rinsed
- 1 onion, diced
- 8 ounces fresh mushrooms, chopped
- 3 cloves garlic, minced
- 1 quart vegetable broth
- 2 cups uncooked quinoa, rinsed
- 1 bunch Swiss chard, stems removed

DIRECTIONS

1. Heat the oil in a large pot over medium heat. Stir in the onion and garlic, and saute 5 minutes, until onion is tender. Mix in quinoa, lentils, and mushrooms. Pour in the broth. Cover, and cook 20 minutes.
2. Remove the pot from heat. Shred chard, and gently mix into the pot. Cover, and allow to sit 5 minutes, or until chard is wilted.

TABBOULEH

Servings: 4 | Prep: 10m | Cooks: 1h | Total: 1h10m

NUTRITION FACTS

Calories: 101 | Carbohydrates: 19.2g | Fat: 3g | Protein: 3.5g | Cholesterol: 0mg

INGREDIENTS

- 1/4 cup bulgur
- 1 onion, finely diced

- 1/2 cup boiling water
- 2 teaspoons olive oil
- 1 cup chopped parsley
- 1 lemon, juiced
- 1/4 cup chopped fresh mint leaves
- salt to taste
- 5 tomatoes, diced

DIRECTIONS

1. Place the bulgur in a small mixing bowl. Add the boiling water, mix and cover with a towel; Let stand for 1 hour. Drain any excess water.
2. Combine the parsley, mint, tomatoes, onion, olive oil, lemon juice and salt. Add the bulgur; mix well and serve.

FRESH TOMATO SALAD
Servings: 7 | Prep: 15m | Cooks: 15m | Total: 30m

NUTRITION FACTS

Calories: 39 | Carbohydrates: 8.6g | Fat: 0.4g | Protein: 1.8g | Cholesterol: 0mg

INGREDIENTS

- 5 tomatoes, diced
- 1/2 cup chopped parsley
- 1 onion, chopped
- 2 tablespoons crushed garlic
- 1 cucumber, sliced
- salt and pepper to taste
- 1 green bell pepper, chopped
- 2 tablespoons white wine vinegar
- 1/2 cup chopped fresh basil

DIRECTIONS

1. In a large bowl, combine the tomato, onion, cucumber, bell pepper, basil, parsley, garlic and vinegar. Toss and add salt and pepper to taste. Chill and serve.

PALEO CHICKEN STEW
Servings: 6 | Prep: 15m | Cooks: 35m | Total: 50m

NUTRITION FACTS

Calories: 145 | Carbohydrates: 20.9g | Fat: 2.5g | Protein: 9.6g | Cholesterol: 21mg

INGREDIENTS

- 2 teaspoons olive oil
- 1 cup fresh spinach, or to taste
- 1 small red onion, chopped
- 1 pinch crushed red pepper, or more to taste
- 2 cloves garlic, minced
- 1 pinch paprika, or more to taste
- 2 skinless, boneless chicken breast halves, cut into cubes
- sea salt to taste
- 2 sweet potatoes, peeled and chopped
- 1/2 cup chicken broth, or more to taste

DIRECTIONS

1. Heat olive oil in a saucepan over medium-high heat. Saute onion and garlic in hot oil until softened, about 5 minutes.
2. Stir chicken, sweet potatoes, spinach, crushed red pepper, paprika, and sea salt with the onion and garlic in the saucepan. Pour as much chicken broth into the saucepan to make the mixture as soup-like or stew-like as you'd like it.
3. Bring the broth to a boil, reduce heat to medium-low, and simmer until the chicken is no longer pink in the middle and the sweet potatoes are tender, about 30 minutes.

EASTER HAM BONE SOUP

Servings: 10 | Prep: 20m | Cooks: 1h55m | Total: 10h15m

NUTRITION FACTS

Calories: 111 | Carbohydrates: 24.8g | Fat: 0.2g | Protein: 3.3g | Cholesterol: 0mg

INGREDIENTS

- 3 quarts water
- 5 green onions, chopped, or more to taste
- 1 ham bone
- 1/2 cup water
- 5 potatoes, cut into 1-inch cubes
- 1/3 cup all-purpose flour
- 4 cups chopped cabbage
- 1 cup light whipping cream
- 2 large stalks celery, chopped

DIRECTIONS

1. Bring 3 quarts water and ham bone to a boil in a large stock pot. Boil until meat from the bone comes off easily, about 1 hour. Remove bone from broth. Allow bone to cool enough to touch; remove as much meat from as possible. Transfer meat to a resealable plastic bag, seal, and refrigerate.
2. Pour broth into a large bowl; cover and refrigerate overnight. Skim and discard any fat from the top of the chilled broth; transfer broth to a large pot.
3. Bring broth to a boil; add potatoes, cabbage, celery, and reserved ham. Continue to simmer until potatoes are tender, about 45 minutes.
4. Whisk 1/2 cup water and flour in a bowl; whisk into potato-ham soup until thickened. Add light cream; stir.

CHICKEN PASTA
Servings: 8 | Prep: 30m | Cooks: 15m | Total: 45m

NUTRITION FACTS

Calories: 185 | Carbohydrates: 26.1g | Fat: 1.8g | Protein: 15.7g | Cholesterol: 27mg

INGREDIENTS

- 3 cups mostaccioli
- 2 tablespoons Italian seasoning
- 3 skinless, boneless chicken breast halves
- 1 (14.5 ounce) can diced tomatoes
- 1/4 onion, chopped
- salt and pepper to taste
- 3 fresh mushrooms, sliced
- 2 tablespoons grated Parmesan cheese

DIRECTIONS

1. Bring a large pot of lightly salted water to a boil. Add pasta and cook for 8 to 10 minutes or until al dente; drain and reserve.
2. Meanwhile, in a large lightly greased skillet over medium heat, cook chicken for about 15 minutes and remove from pan; cool and dice.
3. In a large skillet over medium heat, combine onion, mushrooms, Italian seasoning, tomatoes with juice, salt and pepper; cook until onions are translucent. Remove from heat and add chicken and pasta. Sprinkle Parmesan cheese on top; serve.

BUTTERNUT SQUASH CAJUN FRIES
Servings: 6 | Prep: 20m | Cooks: 25m | Total: 45m

NUTRITION FACTS

Calories: 52 | Carbohydrates: 13.5g | Fat: 0.1g | Protein: 1.2g | Cholesterol: 0mg

INGREDIENTS

- cooking spray
- 1/4 teaspoon ground black pepper, or to taste
- 1 pound butternut squash - peeled, seeded, and cut into thick French fries
- 1/2 teaspoon Cajun seasoning, or to taste
- 1 pinch salt to taste

DIRECTIONS

1. Preheat oven to 450 degrees F (230 degrees C). Spray a baking sheet with cooking spray.
2. Blot any moisture from the butternut squash fries with paper towels, and place on the prepared baking sheet. Sprinkle with salt, black pepper, and Cajun seasoning.
3. Bake in the preheated oven until lightly browned and tender, 15 to 20 minutes, turning once.

CABBAGE ON THE GRILL
Servings: 8 | Prep: 15m | Cooks: 40m | Total: 55m

NUTRITION FACTS

Calories: 41 | Carbohydrates: 9.4g | Fat: 0.2g | Protein: 2.1g | Cholesterol: 0mg

INGREDIENTS

- 1 large head cabbage
- 1 1/2 teaspoons garlic powder, or to taste
- salt and pepper to taste

DIRECTIONS

1. Preheat grill for medium heat.
2. Cut the cabbage into 8 wedges, and remove the core. Place all the wedges on a piece of aluminum foil large enough to wrap the cabbage. Season to taste with garlic powder, salt, and pepper. Seal cabbage in the foil.
3. Grill for 30 to 40 minutes on the preheated grill, until tender.

COUSCOUS WITH MUSHROOMS AND SUN-DRIED TOMATOES
Servings: 4 | Prep: 30m | Cooks: 15m | Total: 45m

NUTRITION FACTS

Calories: 178 | Carbohydrates: 36.1g | Fat: 2g | Protein: 7.5g | Cholesterol: 0mg

INGREDIENTS

- 1 cup dehydrated sun-dried tomatoes
- 1/3 cup fresh basil leaves
- 1 1/2 cups water
- 1/4 cup fresh cilantro, chopped
- 1/2 (10 ounce) package couscous
- 1/2 lemon, juiced
- 1 teaspoon olive oil
- salt and pepper to taste
- 3 cloves garlic, pressed
- 4 ounces portobello mushroom caps, sliced
- 1 bunch green onions, chopped

DIRECTIONS

1. Place the sun-dried tomatoes in a bowl with 1 cup water. Soak 30 minutes, until rehydrated. Drain, reserving water, and chop.
2. In a medium saucepan, combine the reserved sun-dried tomato water with enough water to yield 1 1/2 cups. Bring to a boil. Stir in the couscous. Cover, remove from heat, and allow to sit 5 minutes, until liquid has been absorbed. Gently fluff with a fork.
3. Heat the olive oil in a skillet. Stir in the sun-dried tomatoes, garlic, and green onions. Cook and stir about 5 minutes, until the green onions are tender. Mix in the basil, cilantro, and lemon juice. Season with salt and pepper. Mix in the mushrooms, and continue cooking 3 to 5 minutes. Toss with the cooked couscous to serve.

LENTIL CHILI
Servings: 12 | Prep: 25m | Cooks: 1h | Total: 1h25m

NUTRITION FACTS

Calories: 189 | Carbohydrates: 32.6g | Fat: 3.1g | Protein: 10.9g | Cholesterol: 3mg

INGREDIENTS

- 1 tablespoon olive oil
- 2 tablespoons chili powder
- 1 tablespoon butter
- 1 tablespoon cumin
- 4 cups chopped onion
- 1 dash paprika
- 1 bulb garlic cloves, chopped
- salt to taste
- 1 (16 ounce) package dry lentils

- black pepper to taste
- 1 (6 ounce) can tomato paste
- 2 cups sliced carrots
- 1 (14.5 ounce) can crushed tomatoes
- 2 cups sliced celery
- 2 quarts water

DIRECTIONS

1. Heat the olive oil and melt the butter in a large pot over low heat. Stir in onion and garlic, and cook until tender. Mix in lentils, tomato paste, and crushed tomatoes. Pour in the water. Season chili with chili powder, cumin, paprika, salt, and pepper. Bring to a boil. Reduce heat to low, cover, and simmer 30 minutes, stirring occasionally.
2. Mix carrots and celery into the chili. Continue cooking 20 minutes over low heat, until lentils, carrots, and celery are tender.

MARINATED BEET SALAD

Servings: 4 | Prep: 10m | Cooks: 10m | Total: 4h20m

NUTRITION FACTS

Calories: 89 | Carbohydrates: 21.7g | Fat: 0.2g | Protein: 1.2g | Cholesterol: 0mg

INGREDIENTS

- 1 (16 ounce) can whole beets
- 1/4 cup white wine vinegar
- 1/4 cup white sugar
- 1/4 cup diced red onion
- 1 teaspoon prepared mustard

DIRECTIONS

1. Drain beets, reserving 1/4 cup liquid, and slice into 1/4 to 1/2 inch slivers. Add onions and toss.
2. In a saucepan over medium heat, cook the sugar, mustard and reserved 1/4 cup liquid until dissolved. Add vinegar and bring to boil; remove from heat and allow to cool.
3. Pour over the beet slices and onions, toss and refrigerate for 4 to 6 hours. Remove from refrigerator and serve at room temperature.

CURRIED CUMIN POTATOES

Servings: 8 | Prep: 15m | Cooks: 20m | Total: 35m

NUTRITION FACTS

Calories: 128 | Carbohydrates: 21.4g | Fat: 4g | Protein: 2.7g | Cholesterol: 0mg

INGREDIENTS

- 2 pounds new potatoes, cut into 1/4 inch thick pieces
- 2 teaspoons curry powder
- 2 tablespoons olive oil
- 2 teaspoons coarse sea salt
- 2 tablespoons cumin seed
- 1 teaspoon ground black pepper
- 2 teaspoons ground turmeric
- 3 tablespoons chopped fresh cilantro

DIRECTIONS

1. Place whole potatoes into a saucepan with water to cover. Bring to a boil, and cook until just tender. Drain, and cut potatoes into quarters. Set aside to keep warm.
2. Heat oil in a large saute pan over medium-high heat. Saute the cumin, turmeric, and curry powder for 1 minute. Add potatoes, and saute until toasted. Toss potatoes with sea salt, pepper and fresh cilantro, and serve hot.

TORTILLA SOUP

Servings: 6 | Prep: 20m | Cooks: 50m | Total: 1h10m

NUTRITION FACTS

Calories: 148 | Carbohydrates: 16.5g | Fat: 2.8g | Protein: 14.8g | Cholesterol: 35mg

INGREDIENTS

- 9 cups chicken broth
- 1 teaspoon dried oregano
- 6 cloves roasted garlic
- 1/2 yellow onion, sliced
- 1/2 cup chopped tomatoes
- 2 cups shredded, cooked chicken meat
- 1/2 yellow onion, chopped
- 1 lime, juiced
- 2 fresh jalapeno peppers, sliced into rings
- 6 (6 inch) corn tortillas, cut into strips and toasted for garnish

DIRECTIONS

1. In heavy pot, bring the broth to a boil. Add garlic, tomatoes, chopped onion, jalapeno, and oregano to the stocks. Simmer uncovered for 30 minutes.
2. Broil the sliced onions until soft and a little brown. Add broiled onions, chicken, lime juice to soup, and simmer till chicken is heated.

3. Place toasted tortilla strips in each bowl and pour soup over strips.

PUMPKIN PROTEIN COOKIES

Servings: 14 | Prep: 15m | Cooks: 5m | Total: 20m

NUTRITION FACTS

Calories: 85 | Carbohydrates: 13.1g | Fat: 2.2g | Protein: 4.2g | Cholesterol: 0mg

INGREDIENTS

- 3/4 cup SPLENDA® Granular
- 1 teaspoon ground nutmeg
- 1 cup rolled oats
- 1/2 cup pumpkin puree
- 1 cup whole wheat flour
- 1 tablespoon canola oil
- 1/2 cup soy flour
- 2 teaspoons water
- 1 3/4 teaspoons baking soda
- 2 egg whites
- 1/2 teaspoon baking powder
- 1 teaspoon molasses
- 1/2 teaspoon salt
- 1 tablespoon flax seeds (optional)
- 2 teaspoons ground cinnamon

DIRECTIONS

1. Preheat oven to 350 degrees F (175 degrees C).
2. In a large bowl, whisk together Splenda®, oats, wheat flour, soy flour, baking soda, baking powder, salt, cinnamon, and nutmeg. Stir in pumpkin, canola oil, water, egg whites, and molasses. Stir in flax seeds, if desired. Roll into 14 large balls, and flatten on a baking sheet.
3. Bake for 5 minutes in preheated oven. DO NOT OVERBAKE: the cookies will come out really dry if overbaked.

COLLARD GREENS AND BEANS

Servings: 4 | Prep: 10m | Cooks: 2h25m | Total: 2h35m

NUTRITION FACTS

Calories: 163 | Carbohydrates: 24.8g | Fat: 3.5g | Protein: 8.3g | Cholesterol: 7mg

INGREDIENTS

- 3 slices bacon, coarsely chopped
- 1 tablespoon brown sugar
- 1 red onion, thinly sliced
- 2 teaspoons cider vinegar
- 2 tablespoons minced garlic, or to taste
- 1 teaspoon crushed red pepper flakes, or to taste
- 5 cups collard greens, stems and center ribs discarded and leaves chopped
- salt and black pepper to taste
- 3/4 cup water, or as needed
- 1 (15 ounce) can cannellini beans, drained and rinsed

DIRECTIONS

1. Place the bacon in a large, deep pan with a lid, and cook over medium-high heat, stirring occasionally, until evenly browned, about 10 minutes. Remove the bacon pieces from the pan, and set aside.
2. Reduce the heat to medium-low, and stir the sliced onion into the hot bacon fat. Cook and stir the onion until it begins to brown, scraping the bits off the bottom of the pan, about 8 minutes. Add the garlic, and cook and stir 4 more minutes. Return the bacon to the pan, stir in the collard greens, and toss gently until the greens are wilted, about 3 minutes.
3. Pour in the water to almost cover the collard greens, and stir in the brown sugar, vinegar, crushed red pepper, and salt and pepper. Bring to a boil, cover, reduce heat to low, and simmer the collard greens until very tender, 1 to 2 hours.
4. About 1/2 hour before serving, stir the cannellini beans into the collard greens, and return to a simmer.

BANANA BREAKFAST COOKIES

Servings: 12 | Prep: 10m | Cooks: 20m | Total: 45m | Additional: 15m

NUTRITION FACTS

Calories: 123 | Carbohydrates: 27.4g | Fat: 1.1g | Protein: 2.9g | Cholesterol: 0mg

INGREDIENTS

- 3 very ripe bananas
- 1/3 cup plain yogurt
- 2 cups rolled oats
- 1 teaspoon ground cinnamon
- 1 cup raisins

DIRECTIONS

1. Preheat the oven to 350 degrees F (175 degrees C). Line cookie sheets with parchment paper.

2. Mash bananas in a large bowl. Add oats, raisins, yogurt, and cinnamon. Mix well and allow to sit for 15 minutes.
3. Drop spoonfuls of dough 2 inches apart onto the prepared cookie sheets.
4. Bake in the preheated oven until lightly browned, about 20 minutes.

TRAIL MIX COOKIES
Servings: 36 | Prep: 20m | Cooks: 10m | Total: 30m

NUTRITION FACTS

Calories: 77 | Carbohydrates: 14.1g | Fat: 2g | Protein: 1.4g | Cholesterol: 0mg

INGREDIENTS

- 1/2 cup applesauce
- 1/2 teaspoon salt
- 1/2 cup white sugar
- 3/4 teaspoon ground cinnamon
- 1/2 cup brown sugar
- 1 1/4 cups quick cooking oats
- 1 1/2 teaspoons vanilla extract
- 1/2 cup semisweet chocolate chips
- 2 egg whites
- 1/2 cup chopped walnuts
- 1 1/4 cups all-purpose flour
- 1/3 cup dried cranberries
- 1 teaspoon baking soda

DIRECTIONS

1. Preheat oven to 350 degrees F (175 degrees C). Grease 2 baking sheets.
2. Beat applesauce, white sugar, brown sugar, and vanilla in a large bowl. In another bowl, use an electric mixer to beat egg whites until they are frothy and begin to firm up. Fold egg whites into applesauce mixture. Combine the flour, baking soda, salt, and cinnamon. Fold into the egg mixture. Stir in the oats, chocolate chips, walnuts, and cranberries. Drop by heaping teaspoons on prepared baking sheets.
3. Bake cookies in preheated oven until set and lightly browned, about 10 minutes. Remove immediately to wire racks to cool.

SPLIT PEA SOUP WITHOUT PORK
Servings: 10 | Prep: 15m | Cooks: 2h | Total: 2h15m

NUTRITION FACTS

Calories: 65 | Carbohydrates: 11.2g | Fat: 0.3g | Protein: 4.8g | Cholesterol: 0mg

INGREDIENTS

- 1 pound dried split peas
- 2 (14.5 ounce) cans low-fat, low sodium chicken broth
- 1 stalk celery, diced
- 3 cups water
- 2 large carrots, peeled and diced
- salt and pepper to taste

DIRECTIONS

1. Rinse and pick through peas. Place them in a large pot with the celery, carrots, broth and water. Bring to a boil, then reduce heat, cover and simmer until peas have fallen apart, 1 to 2 hours. Season with salt and pepper before serving.

SLOW COOKER PUMPKIN STEEL CUT OATS
Servings: 8 | Prep: 5m | Cooks: 6h | Total: 6h5m

NUTRITION FACTS

Calories: 195 | Carbohydrates: 38.2g | Fat: 2.9g | Protein: 5.9g | Cholesterol: 0mg

INGREDIENTS

- cooking spray (such as Pam®)
- 1 cup brown sugar replacement (such as Splenda® Brown Sugar Blend)
- 6 cups water
- 2 tablespoons ground cinnamon
- 1 (15 ounce) can pumpkin puree
- 1 tablespoon pumpkin pie spice
- 1 1/2 cups steel-cut oats

DIRECTIONS

1. Prepare the crock of your slow cooker with cooking spray.
2. Stir water, pumpkin puree, oats, brown sugar replacement, cinnamon, and pumpkin pie spice together in the prepared slow cooker.
3. Cook on Low for 6 hours. Stir before serving.

QUINOA PORRIDGE
Servings: 3 | Prep: 5m | Cooks: 30m | Total: 35m

NUTRITION FACTS

Calories: 173 | Carbohydrates: 31.3g | Fat: 3g | Protein: 4.3g | Cholesterol: 0mg

INGREDIENTS

- 1/2 cup quinoa
- 2 tablespoons brown sugar
- 1/4 teaspoon ground cinnamon
- 1 teaspoon vanilla extract (optional)
- 1 1/2 cups almond milk
- 1 pinch salt
- 1/2 cup water

DIRECTIONS

1. Heat a saucepan over medium heat and measure in the quinoa. Season with cinnamon and cook until toasted, stirring frequently, about 3 minutes. Pour in the almond milk, water and vanilla and stir in the brown sugar and salt. Bring to a boil, then cook over low heat until the porridge is thick and grains are tender, about 25 minutes. Add more water if needed if the liquid has dried up before it finishes cooking. Stir occasionally, especially at the end, to prevent burning.

BANANA OAT ENERGY BARS
Servings: 12 | Prep: 15m | Cooks: 20m | Total: 35m

NUTRITION FACTS

Calories: 124 | Carbohydrates: 20g | Fat: 4g | Protein: 3.6g | Cholesterol: 0mg

INGREDIENTS

- 2 cups rolled oats
- 1 apple, grated
- 2 bananas, mashed
- 1 cup unsweetened applesauce
- 2 carrots, grated
- 1/2 cup chopped peanuts

DIRECTIONS

1. Preheat oven to 350 degrees F (175 degrees C). Grease a 9x13-inch baking dish.
2. Mix oats, bananas, carrots, apple, applesauce, and peanuts together in a bowl; spread into the prepared baking dish.
3. Bake in the preheated oven until golden brown, about 20 minutes.

RAW HUMMUS

Servings: 20 | Prep: 15m | Cooks: 2m | Total: 3d17m

NUTRITION FACTS

Calories: 67 | Carbohydrates: 10.8g | Fat: 1.8g | Protein: 3.3g | Cholesterol: 0mg

INGREDIENTS

- 1 1/2 cups dry garbanzo beans
- 4 cloves garlic, crushed or to taste
- 2 tablespoons tahini
- 1 cup filtered or spring water
- 1 teaspoon sea salt
- 1 pinch paprika
- 2 lemons, juiced

DIRECTIONS

1. Soak the beans for 24 hours. Drain, and let sit for 2 to 3 days, until the bean's sprouts are about 1/2 inch long. Rinse the beans once or twice a day.
2. Bring a large pot of water to a boil. Remove from heat, and let stand for 1 minute. Place the sprouted beans in the hot water, and let sit for 1 minute. Drain. If you do not do this step, the hummus will be awful.
3. Place the sprouted beans into the container of a large food processor. Add the tahini, sea salt, lemon juice, and garlic. Process until smooth, adding water if necessary. It will take 3 to 5 minutes to blend. Let sit in the food processor for 5 minutes to allow the beans to absorb as much of the water as possible. If too thick, add more water, and blend again. Taste and adjust seasonings if needed. Spoon into a serving dish, and garnish with paprika.

SUPER EASY SLOW COOKER CHICKEN ENCHILADA MEAT

Servings: 10 | Prep: 15m | Cooks: 8h | Total: 8h15m

NUTRITION FACTS

Calories: 93 | Carbohydrates: 8.8g | Fat: 1.8g | Protein: 10.4g | Cholesterol: 23mg

INGREDIENTS

- 2 cups chicken broth
- 2 teaspoons ground cumin
- 1 (14.5 ounce) can diced tomatoes
- 1 teaspoon oregano
- 1/3 cup chili powder

- 1 teaspoon salt, or to taste
- 1/2 cup all-purpose flour
- 1 pinch cayenne pepper, or more to taste (optional)
- 1 clove garlic
- 4 skinless, boneless chicken breast halves

DIRECTIONS

1. Blend chicken broth, tomatoes, chili powder, flour, garlic, cumin, oregano, salt, and cayenne pepper in a blender until smooth.
2. Put chicken breast in bottom of a slow cooker; pour blended enchilada sauce over the chicken.
3. Cook on Low 8 to 9 hours (or 4 to 6 hours on High). Shred the chicken with 2 large forks and stir into the sauce.

ITALIAN STEWED TOMATOES
Servings: 9 | Prep: 30m | Cooks: 10m | Total: 40m

NUTRITION FACTS

Calories: 100 | Carbohydrates: 22.2g | Fat: 1g | Protein: 4.6g | Cholesterol: 0mg

INGREDIENTS

- 24 large tomatoes - peeled, seeded and chopped
- 1/4 cup chopped green bell pepper
- 1 cup chopped celery
- 2 teaspoons dried basil
- 1/2 cup chopped onion
- 1 tablespoon white sugar

DIRECTIONS

1. In a large saucepan over medium heat, combine tomatoes, celery, onion, bell pepper, basil and sugar. Cover and cook for 10 minutes, stirring occasionally to prevent sticking.

CURRIED LENTILS
Servings: 2 | Prep: 20m | Cooks: 20m | Total: 40m

NUTRITION FACTS

Calories: 145 | Carbohydrates: 25.2g | Fat: 0.5g | Protein: 10.8g | Cholesterol: 0mg

INGREDIENTS

- 1/2 cup dried lentils
- 1 tablespoon curry paste
- 1 cup water
- salt to taste
- 3/4 cup canned cream of coconut

DIRECTIONS

1. Rinse lentils and place in a saucepan with the water. Bring to a boil, then cover, and simmer over low heat for 15 minutes. Stir in the curry paste, coconut cream and season with salt to taste. Return to a simmer, and cook for an additional 10 to 15 minutes, until tender.

ALL-STAR VEGGIE BURGER
Servings: 8 | Prep: 20m | Cooks: 10m | Total: 30m

NUTRITION FACTS

Calories: 161 | Carbohydrates: 23.8g | Fat: 4.7g | Protein: 8.3g | Cholesterol: 0mg

INGREDIENTS

- 1 (15.5 ounce) can garbanzo beans, drained and mashed
- 5 tablespoons Korean barbeque sauce
- 8 fresh basil leaves, chopped
- 1/2 teaspoon salt
- 1/4 cup oat bran
- 1/2 teaspoon ground black pepper
- 1/4 cup quick cooking oats
- 3/4 teaspoon garlic powder
- 1 cup cooked brown rice
- 3/4 teaspoon dried sage
- 1 (14 ounce) package firm tofu
- 2 teaspoons vegetable oil

DIRECTIONS

1. In a large bowl, stir together the mashed garbanzo beans and basil. Mix in the oat bran, quick oats, and rice; the mixture should seem a little dry.
2. In a separate bowl, mash the tofu with your hands, trying to squeeze out as much of the water as possible. Drain of the water, and repeat the process until there is hardly any water worth pouring off. It is not necessary to remove all of the water. Pour the barbeque sauce over the tofu, and stir to coat.
3. Stir the tofu into the garbanzo beans and oats. Season with salt, pepper, garlic powder, and sage; mix until well blended.
4. Heat the oil in a large skillet over medium-high heat. Form patties out of the bean mixture, and fry them in hot oil for about 5 minutes per side. Serve as you would burgers.

CHILLED CANTALOUPE SOUP

Servings: 6 | Prep: 20m | Cooks: 1h | Total: 1h20m

NUTRITION FACTS

Calories: 69 | Carbohydrates: 16.4g | Fat: 0.3g | Protein: 1.4g | Cholesterol: 0mg

INGREDIENTS

- 1 cantaloupe - peeled, seeded and cubed
- 1 tablespoon fresh lime juice
- 2 cups orange juice
- 1/4 teaspoon ground cinnamon

DIRECTIONS

1. Peel, seed, and cube the cantaloupe.
2. Place cantaloupe and 1/2 cup orange juice in a blender or food processor; cover, and process until smooth. Transfer to large bowl. Stir in lime juice, cinnamon, and remaining orange juice. Cover, and refrigerate for at least one hour. Garnish with mint if desired.

WHITE BEANS AND PEPPERS

Servings: 4 | Prep: 10m | Cooks: 15m | Total: 25m

NUTRITION FACTS

Calories: 150 | Carbohydrates: 26.6g | Fat: 1.8g | Protein: 8.5g | Cholesterol: 0mg

INGREDIENTS

- 1 teaspoon olive oil
- 1 pinch dried oregano
- 1/4 large onion, chopped
- ground cayenne pepper to taste
- 1 yellow gypsy (bull horn) sweet pepper, chopped
- salt to taste
- 1 (15 ounce) can great Northern beans, drained
- ground black pepper to taste

DIRECTIONS

1. Heat the oil in a skillet over medium heat. Stir in onion and sweet pepper, and cook until tender. Mix in beans. Season with oregano, cayenne pepper, salt, and black pepper. Continue cooking, stirring occasionally, until beans are heated through.

PARSLEY POTATOES

Servings: 6 | Prep: 15m | Cooks: 15m | Total: 30m

NUTRITION FACTS

Calories: 134 | Carbohydrates: 23.5g | Fat: 2.9g | Protein: 4.3g | Cholesterol: <1mg

INGREDIENTS

- 1 1/2 pounds new red potatoes
- 1 cup chicken broth
- 1 tablespoon vegetable oil
- 1 cup chopped fresh parsley
- 1 onion, chopped
- 1/2 teaspoon ground black pepper
- 1 clove garlic, crushed
- 1/2 teaspoon lemon pepper

DIRECTIONS

1. Peel a strip of skin from around the center of each potato, place the potatoes in cold water. Set aside.
2. Heat oil in a large skillet over medium high heat. Saute onion and garlic for 5 minutes or until tender. Pour in broth and 3/4 cup of the parsley; mix well. Bring to a boil.
3. Place the potatoes into a large pot full of salted water. Bring the water to a boil; then reduce heat. Simmer covered, for 10 minutes or until the potatoes are tender.
4. Remove potatoes with a slotted spoon to a serving bowl. Sprinkle the black pepper into the skillet and stir.. Pour the peppered sauce over potatoes and sprinkle with remaining parsley.

PUMPKIN PIE FOR DIETERS

Servings: 6 | Prep: 10m | Cooks: 1h | Total: 1h10m | Additional: 1h

NUTRITION FACTS

Calories: 110 | Carbohydrates: 23g | Fat: 0.3g | Protein: 1.5g | Cholesterol: 0mg

INGREDIENTS

- 1 (15 ounce) can pumpkin puree
- 1 teaspoon pumpkin pie spice
- 1/2 cup skim milk
- 1 (8 ounce) container fat free frozen whipped topping
- 1 (1 ounce) package instant sugar-free vanilla pudding mix
- 1/2 teaspoon lemon pepper

DIRECTIONS

1. In a medium bowl, mix together the pumpkin, milk, and instant pudding mix. Stir in the pumpkin pie spice, and fold in half of the whipped topping.
2. Pour into an 8-inch pie plate, and spread remaining whipped topping over the top. Chill for 1 hour, or until set.

SLOW COOKER CIDER APPLESAUCE

Servings: 16 | Prep: 10m | Cooks: 4h | Total: 4h10m

NUTRITION FACTS

Calories: 76 | Carbohydrates: 20.2g | Fat: 0.3g | Protein: 0.4g | Cholesterol: 0mg

INGREDIENTS

- pounds apples - peeled, cored, and thinly sliced
- 1/2 teaspoon ground cloves
- 1 1/2 tablespoons ground cinnamon
- 1/4 teaspoon ground nutmeg

DIRECTIONS

1. Layer apples into a slow cooker. Sprinkle cinnamon, cloves, and nutmeg over the apples.
2. Cook on High until apples are soft, 4 to 5 hours. Whisk apples vigorously for a chunkier-style applesauce. Puree with an immersion blender for a smoother applesauce.

SHREDDED POTATO SALMON CAKES

Servings: 12 | Prep: 25m | Cooks: 6m | Total: 31m

NUTRITION FACTS

Calories: 139 | Carbohydrates: 15.9g | Fat: 4.6g | Protein: 8.7g | Cholesterol: 42mg

INGREDIENTS

- 3 medium potatoes, peeled and shredded
- 2 tablespoons capers, drained
- 2 eggs
- 1 red bell pepper, seeded and chopped
- salt and pepper to taste
- 3/4 cup chopped canned banana peppers
- 1 teaspoon Italian seasoning
- 3/4 cup sliced fresh mushrooms
- 1/2 pound cooked flaked salmon
- 3/4 cup dry bread crumbs

- 3 green onions, chopped
- 1 cup oil for frying, or as needed

DIRECTIONS

1. Squeeze as much liquid from the potatoes as you can, and place in a large bowl. Beat the eggs with salt, pepper, and Italian seasoning, and mix with the potatoes. Mix in salmon, green onions, capers, red bell pepper, banana peppers, mushrooms and bread crumbs. Form into about 12 patties about 3/4 inch thick.
2. Heat 1/4 inch of oil in a large heavy skillet over medium-high heat. Fry the patties for about 3 minutes per side, or until golden brown. Drain on paper towels quickly before serving. Try to fry all the patties at one time, otherwise the mixture becomes stiff.

EASY SPICED BROWN RICE WITH CORN
Servings: 6 | Prep: 5m | Cooks: 1h | Total: 1h5m

NUTRITION FACTS

Calories: 133 | Carbohydrates: 24.4g | Fat: 3.2g | Protein: 2.7g | Cholesterol: 0mg

INGREDIENTS

- 2 cups water
- 1 cup frozen corn kernels
- 1 cup brown rice
- 1/2 teaspoon dried cilantro
- 1 tablespoon olive oil
- 1/2 teaspoon cumin seed
- 1/2 teaspoon salt

DIRECTIONS

1. In a saucepan, mix the water, rice, olive oil, and salt, and bring to a boil. Mix in the corn, cilantro, and cumin. Reduce heat, cover, and simmer 45 to 60 minutes, until the liquid has been absorbed.

BLACK BEAN AND RICE SALAD
Servings: 8 | Prep: 10m | Cooks: 10m | Total: 20m

NUTRITION FACTS

Calories: 140 | Carbohydrates: 28g | Fat: 2.8g | Protein: 3.5g | Cholesterol: 0mg

INGREDIENTS

- 2 tomatoes, chopped

- 1 (15 ounce) can whole kernel corn; drain and reserve liquid
- 1 large red bell pepper, chopped
- 1 (15 ounce) can black beans; drain and reserve liquid
- 2 jalapeno peppers, minced
- 1 tablespoon olive oil
- 3/4 cup lemon juice
- 1/2 cup chopped onion
- 1 1/4 teaspoons dried cilantro
- 1/2 teaspoon minced garlic
- 1/4 teaspoon dried basil
- 1 1/2 cups instant brown rice
- /8 teaspoon red pepper flakes
- salt and pepper to taste

DIRECTIONS

1. In a large bowl, combine tomatoes, red bell pepper, jalapeno pepper, lemon juice, cilantro, basil, red pepper flakes, corn, and beans. Stir to combine the vegetables, then set aside.
2. In a medium saucepan, heat olive oil at a medium-low heat. Add onions and saute until they are translucent. Add garlic and saute for another minute. Pour in rice and toss to coat. Add reserved liquid from the corn and beans, along with any additional liquid as directed on the rice box. Cook the rice to package specifications. Let the rice cool slightly.
3. Combine the rice and vegetable mixture. Salt and pepper to taste and serve.

SLOW COOKER ROOT VEGETABLE TAGINE
Servings: 8 | Prep: 50m | Cooks: 9h | Total: 9h50m

NUTRITION FACTS

Calories: 131 | Carbohydrates: 31g | Fat: 0.7g | Protein: 2.8g | Cholesterol: 0mg

INGREDIENTS

- 1 pound parsnips, peeled and diced
- 1 teaspoon ground cumin
- 1 pound turnips, peeled and diced
- 1/2 teaspoon ground ginger
- 2 medium onions, chopped
- 1/2 teaspoon ground cinnamon
- 1 pound carrots, peeled and diced
- 1/4 teaspoon ground cayenne pepper
- 6 dried apricots, chopped
- 1 tablespoon dried parsley
- 4 pitted prunes, chopped

- 1 tablespoon dried cilantro
- 1 teaspoon ground turmeric
- 1 (14 ounce) can vegetable broth

DIRECTIONS

1. In a slow cooker, toss together the parsnips, turnips, onions, carrots, apricots, and prunes. Season with turmeric, cumin, ginger, cinnamon, cayenne pepper, parsley, and cilantro. Pour in the vegetable broth.
2. Cover, and cook 9 hours on Low.

RUSH HOUR REFRIED BEANS

Servings: 4 | Prep: 10m | Cooks: 10m | Total: 20m

NUTRITION FACTS

Calories: 68 | Carbohydrates: 12.1g | Fat: 0.6g | Protein: 3.7g | Cholesterol: 0mg

INGREDIENTS

- 2 tablespoons bacon grease
- 1 (15 ounce) can pinto beans, undrained
- 2 tablespoons chopped onion
- 1/4 teaspoon ground cumin
- 1 teaspoon minced garlic

DIRECTIONS

3. Heat bacon grease in a skillet over medium heat. Cook and stir onion and garlic in the hot bacon grease until onions are softened, 5 to 7 minutes. Mash pinto beans and cumin into onion mixture using a potato masher until reaching your desired consistency. Cook and stir bean mixture until heated through, 3 to 5 minutes.

HOMEMADE SAUERKRAUT

Servings: 8 | Prep: 10m | Cooks: 15m | Total: 25m

NUTRITION FACTS

Calories: 45 | Carbohydrates: 10.2g | Fat: 0.2g | Protein: 2.1g | Cholesterol: 0mg

INGREDIENTS

- 1 cup water
- 1/2 teaspoon celery seed
- 1 cup distilled white vinegar, divided

- 1/2 teaspoon onion powder
- 1/2 onion, diced
- 1/2 teaspoon garlic powder
- 1 head cabbage, cored and shredded
- ground black pepper to taste
- 3/4 teaspoon sea salt

DIRECTIONS

1. Combine water, 1/2 of the vinegar, and onion in a pot over high heat; add cabbage, sea salt, celery seed, onion powder, garlic powder, and black pepper. Pour the remaining vinegar over cabbage mixture. Cover pot and bring water to a boil; cook mixture for about 3 minutes.
2. Stir cabbage mixture and return lid to pot; cook, stirring occasionally, until cabbage is tender and wilted, 10 to 15 minutes more.

CARYN'S CHICKEN

Servings: 4 | Prep: 10m | Cooks: 10m | Total: 20m

NUTRITION FACTS

Calories: 250 | Carbohydrates: 29.9g | Fat: 3.1g | Protein: 27g | Cholesterol: 0mg

INGREDIENTS

- 4 skinless, boneless chicken breast halves - pounded thin
- 3 tablespoons thinly sliced green onion
- 6 oranges, juiced
- ground black pepper to taste

DIRECTIONS

1. Hit the chicken fillets with a tenderizing mallet until they are slightly thinned out.
2. Put the orange juice, green onions and black pepper into a skillet over medium heat. Don't cook over high heat, or the juice will burn and go bitter.
3. Poach the chicken in the juice mixture until it is firm and the juices run clear. This usually takes about 10 minutes, depending on the thickness of the filets. Place the chicken on a serving plate and pour some of the juice mixture on top. Serve.

BREAKFAST BROWNIES

Servings: 12 | Prep: 15m | Cooks: 20m | Total: 40m | Additional: 5m

NUTRITION FACTS

Calories: 129 | Carbohydrates: 20.9g | Fat: 4.1g | Protein: 3.3g | Cholesterol: 16mg

INGREDIENTS

- 1 1/2 cups quick-cooking oats
- 1/4 teaspoon salt
- 3/4 cup brown sugar
- 1 banana, mashed
- 3/4 cup flax seed meal
- 1/4 cup rice milk
- 1/2 cup gluten-free all purpose baking flour
- 1 egg
- 1 teaspoon baking powder
- 1 teaspoon vanilla extract
- 1/2 teaspoon ground cinnamon

DIRECTIONS

1. Preheat oven to 350 degrees F (175 degrees C). Lightly grease an 8x10-inch baking pan.
2. Mix oats, brown sugar, flax seed meal, flour, baking powder, cinnamon, and salt together in a bowl. Mix banana, rice milk, egg, and vanilla extract together in a separate bowl. Pour banana mixture into flour mixture; stir to combine. Pour batter into the prepared baking pan.
3. Bake brownies in the preheated oven until a toothpick inserted in the center comes out clean, about 20 minutes. Cover pan with a towel to hold in moisture and cool brownies for at least 5 minutes before serving.

BBQ CORN

Servings: 10 | Prep: 10m | Cooks: 2h | Total: 10h10m

NUTRITION FACTS

Calories: 121 | Carbohydrates: 20.7g | Fat: 1.1g | Protein: 3.4g | Cholesterol: 0mg

INGREDIENTS

- 10 ears fresh corn with husks
- 1 (7 pound) bag of ice cubes
- 1 quart beer

DIRECTIONS

1. Place whole ears of corn in an ice chest. Pour beer over top. Dump ice out over the ears of corn. Place the lid on the cooler, and let sit 8 hours, or overnight.
2. Preheat smoker to 250 degrees F (120 degrees C).

3. Place corn in the smoker and close the lid. Cook for 1 to 2 hours, turning every 20 minutes or so. Kernels should give easily under pressure when done. To eat, just peel back the husks and use them for a handle.

GINGERY CARROT SALAD
Servings: 6 | Prep: 20m | Cooks: 25m | Total: 45m

NUTRITION FACTS

Calories: 136 | Carbohydrates: 26.4g | Fat: 3.8g | Protein: 1.6g | Cholesterol: 0mg

INGREDIENTS

- 1 pound carrots, cut diagonally into thin slices
- 1/4 teaspoon cinnamon
- 2 tablespoons cider vinegar
- 1 teaspoon grated fresh ginger
- 1 tablespoon olive oil
- 1/8 teaspoon seasoned salt
- 2 tablespoons Splenda
- 1 dash cayenne pepper
- 1 clove garlic, grated
- 1/2 cup raisins
- 1/4 teaspoon ground cumin

DIRECTIONS

1. Bring a large pot of water to boil. Add carrots, and continue to boil until just tender, about 2 minutes. Rinse with cold water, drain well, and set aside.
2. In a large bowl, whisk together the vinegar, olive oil, Splenda, and garlic. Season with cumin, cinnamon, ginger, salt, and cayenne pepper. Stir in carrots and raisins, and toss with dressing. Cover, and refrigerate at least 4 hours.

SLOW COOKER CHICKEN CURRY WITH QUINOA
Servings: 6 | Prep: 30m | Cooks: 4m | Total: 4h30m

NUTRITION FACTS

Calories: 185 | Carbohydrates: 14.4g | Fat: 3.1g | Protein: 24.4g | Cholesterol: 59mg

INGREDIENTS

- 1 1/2 pounds diced chicken breast meat
- 1/4 cup nonfat milk

- 3/4 cup chopped onion
- 1 tablespoon curry powder
- 1 1/4 cups chopped celery
- 1/4 teaspoon paprika
- 13/4 cups chopped Granny Smith apples
- 1/3 cup quinoa
- 1 cup chicken broth

DIRECTIONS

1. Place the chicken, onion, celery, apple, chicken broth, milk, curry powder, and paprika into a slow cooker; stir until mixed. Cover, and cook on Low for 4 to 5 hours. Stir in the quinoa during the final 35 minutes of cooking. Serve when quinoa is tender.

OKRA WITH TOMATOES
Servings: 6 | Prep: 15m | Cooks: 15m | Total: 30m

NUTRITION FACTS

Calories: 66 | Carbohydrates: 13.1g | Fat: 1.1g | Protein: 2.8g | Cholesterol: 0mg

INGREDIENTS

- 1 teaspoon olive oil
- 1 pound frozen sliced okra
- 3 cloves garlic, minced
- 1 (8 ounce) can canned diced tomatoes
- 1 small onion, minced
- 1 (15 ounce) can stewed tomatoes
- 1 teaspoon cayenne pepper
- salt and ground black pepper to taste
- 1/2 green bell pepper, minced

DIRECTIONS

1. Cover the bottom of a skillet with the olive oil and place over medium heat. Place the garlic, onion, and cayenne pepper in the skillet and stir until fragrant. Stir in the green pepper. Cook and stir until tender, about 5 minutes. Stir in the frozen okra and allow to cook for 5 minutes more. Stir in both the diced and the stewed tomatoes. Season with salt and pepper. Reduce heat to medium-low and simmer until all vegetables are tender, 5 to 7 minutes.

SLOW COOKER CARROT CAKE STEEL CUT OATS
Servings: 16 | Prep: 10m | Cooks: 6h | Total: 6h10m

NUTRITION FACTS

Calories: 139 | Carbohydrates: 30.1g | Fat: 1.4g | Protein: 3.1g | Cholesterol: 0mg

INGREDIENTS

- 10 cups water
- 1 cup raisins
- 23 ounces unsweetened applesauce
- 1/3 cup granular no-calorie sucralose sweetener (such as Splenda®) (optional)
- 2 cups steel cut oats
- 2 tablespoons ground cinnamon
- 1 (10 ounce) bag shredded carrots
- 1 tablespoon pumpkin pie spice
- 1 (8 ounce) can crushed pineapple, drained
- 1 teaspoon salt (optional)

DIRECTIONS

1. Combine water, applesauce, oats, carrots, pineapple, raisins, sweetener, cinnamon, pumpkin pie spice, and salt in the crock of a 7-quart or larger slow cooker.
2. Cook on Low for 6 hours.

CB'S BLACK EYED PEAS

Servings: 10 | Prep: 15m | Cooks: 4h10m | Total: 4h25m

NUTRITION FACTS

Calories: 168 | Carbohydrates: 26.1g | Fat: 2.5g | Protein: 11.2g | Cholesterol: 4mg

INGREDIENTS

- 4 slices bacon, chopped
- 1 jalapeno pepper, finely chopped
- 1 pound dry black-eyed peas
- 1 clove garlic, minced
- 6 cups water
- 1 tablespoon chili powder
- 1 onion, chopped
- salt to taste
- 1 (14.5 ounce) can diced tomatoes, undrained
- 1/2 teaspoon lemon pepper

DIRECTIONS

1. Place the bacon in a large, deep skillet, and cook over medium heat, stirring occasionally, until evenly browned, about 10 minutes.
2. Place the dried peas, water, onion, tomatoes, jalapeno pepper, garlic, and chili powder into a slow cooker, and stir to combine. Stir in the bacon and bacon grease, and set the cooker on High. Cook until peas are tender, about 4 hours. Season to taste with salt, and serve.

ROASTED EGGPLANT AND MUSHROOMS
Servings: 2 | Prep: 10m | Cooks: 45m | Total: 55m

NUTRITION FACTS

Calories: 118 | Carbohydrates: 25.8g | Fat: 1.1g | Protein: 6.6g | Cholesterol: 0mg

INGREDIENTS

- 1 medium eggplant, peeled and cubed
- 1/2 cup water
- 2 small zucchini, cubed
- 1 clove garlic, minced
- 1/2 small yellow onion, chopped
- 1/2 teaspoon dried basil
- 1 (8 ounce) package mushrooms, sliced
- salt and pepper to taste
- 1 1/2 tablespoons tomato paste

DIRECTIONS

1. Preheat oven to 450 degrees F (230 degrees C).
2. Place eggplant, zucchini, onion and mushrooms in a 2 quart casserole dish. In a small bowl combine the tomato paste with the water, and stir in garlic, basil, salt and pepper. Pour over the vegetables and mix well.
3. Bake in preheated oven for 45 minutes, or until eggplant is tender, stirring occasionally. Add water as necessary if vegetables begin to stick; however, vegetables should be fairly dry, with slightly browned edges.

CITRUS BROILED ALASKA SALMON
Servings: 8 | Prep: 15m | Cooks: 15m | Total: 30m

NUTRITION FACTS

Calories: 168 | Carbohydrates: 11.6g | Fat: 3.9g | Protein: 21.5g | Cholesterol: 0mg

INGREDIENTS

- 4 large oranges

- 1/2 cup chopped green onions
- 8 (4 ounce) fillets salmon
- 2 teaspoons cracked black pepper
- 2 teaspoons red wine vinegar

DIRECTIONS

1. Preheat the oven's broiler.
2. Slice, peel, and pith oranges; slice crosswise into 1/4 inch rounds. Season fillets with salt. Place salmon fillets on broiling pan.
3. Place the pan of fillets 4 to 6 inches from heat. Cook for 15 minutes under the preheated broiler, or 10 minutes per inch of thickness. Remove from broiler just before they are cooked through. Sprinkle with vinegar. Arrange orange rounds on top. Sprinkle with green onions and cracked black pepper. Broil 1 minute longer.

CHOCOLATE-BANANA TOFU PUDDING

Servings: 4 | Prep: 10m | Cooks: 1h | Total: 1h10m | Additional: 1h

NUTRITION FACTS

Calories: 124 | Carbohydrates: 21.2g | Fat: 3.5g | Protein: 6.1g | Cholesterol: 0mg

INGREDIENTS

- 1 banana, broken into chunks
- 5 tablespoons unsweetened cocoa powder
- 1 (12 ounce) package soft silken tofu
- 3 tablespoons soy milk
- 1/4 cup confectioners' sugar
- 1 pinch ground cinnamon

DIRECTIONS

1. Place the banana, tofu, sugar, cocoa powder, soy milk, and cinnamon into a blender. Cover, and puree until smooth. Pour into individual serving dishes, and refrigerate for 1 hour before serving.

BAR-B-Q BAKED BEANS

Servings: 14 | Prep: 10m | Cooks: 1h | Total: 1h10m

NUTRITION FACTS

Calories: 166 | Carbohydrates: 27g | Fat: 3.3g | Protein: 7.3g | Cholesterol: 5mg

INGREDIENTS

- 1 (15 ounce) can kidney beans, drained (optional)
- 2 tablespoons brown sugar
- 1 (15 ounce) can pinto beans, drained
- 1 tablespoon Dijon mustard
- 1 (15 ounce) can lima beans, drained
- 1 tablespoon Worcestershire sauce
- 1 (16 ounce) can great Northern beans, drained
- 2 tablespoons molasses
- 1 (12 ounce) bottle chili sauce
- 3 slices bacon, cut in half

DIRECTIONS

1. Preheat oven to 325 degrees F (165 degrees C).
2. In a medium baking dish, mix kidney beans, pinto beans, lima beans, great northern beans, chili sauce, brown sugar, Dijon mustard, Worcestershire sauce and molasses. Top with bacon.
3. Bake 1 hour in the preheated oven, until thick and bubbly.

SWEET CARROT SALAD

Servings: 8 | Prep: 10m | Cooks: 30m | Total: 40m

NUTRITION FACTS

Calories: 105 | Carbohydrates: 20.6g | Fat: 2.9g | Protein: 1g | Cholesterol: 1mg

INGREDIENTS

- 1 pound carrots, grated
- 1 tablespoon honey
- 1 cup crushed pineapple
- 2 tablespoons mayonnaise, or to taste
- 1/2 cup raisins
- 1 dash lemon juice

DIRECTIONS

1. In a large bowl, mix together the carrots, pineapple and raisins. Stir in the honey, mayonnaise and lemon juice until evenly coated. Refrigerate for at least 30 minutes before serving to let the flavors meld.

FLORENTINE TOMATO SOUP

Servings: 5 | Prep: 10m | Cooks: 15m | Total: 25m

NUTRITION FACTS

Calories: 54 | Carbohydrates: 8g | Fat: 1.3g | Protein: 3.2g | Cholesterol: < 1mg

INGREDIENTS

- 1 teaspoon olive oil
- 1 1/2 cups water
- 1/2 cup chopped green bell pepper
- 1 tablespoon minced fresh basil
- 1/2 cup chopped onion
- 1 teaspoon chicken bouillon granules
- 1 clove garlic, minced
- 1/4 teaspoon ground black pepper
- 1 (14.5 ounce) can diced tomatoes
- 1 (10 ounce) package frozen chopped spinach, thawed

DIRECTIONS

1. In a large saucepan over medium heat, cook bell pepper, onion and garlic in oil until tender. Stir in tomatoes, water, basil, bouillon and black pepper. Bring to a boil, then reduce heat and simmer 10 minutes.
2. Stir in spinach and cook 5 to 7 minutes more.

ROASTED GRAPES AND CARROTS
Servings: 8 | Prep: 5m | Cooks: 15m | Total: 20m

NUTRITION FACTS

Calories: 140 | Carbohydrates: 26.9g | Fat: 4.2g | Protein: 1.5g | Cholesterol: 0mg

INGREDIENTS

- 2 pounds red seedless grapes
- 2 tablespoons olive oil
- 1 (16 ounce) package peeled, baby carrots
- 1 teaspoon ground cumin
- 1 medium red onion, cut into wedges

DIRECTIONS

1. Preheat oven to 375 degrees F (190 degrees C). Line a baking sheet with aluminum foil.

2. Toss together the grapes, carrots, and red onion in olive oil to coat. Sprinkle with cumin and toss to evenly distribute. Spread mixture on baking sheet.
3. Roast in preheated oven until carrots have begun to soften, about 15 to 20 minutes.

FLORENTINE TOMATO SOUP
Servings: 5 | Prep: 10m | Cooks: 15m | Total: 25m

NUTRITION FACTS

Calories: 54 | Carbohydrates: 8g | Fat: 1.3g | Protein: 3.2g | Cholesterol: < 1mg

INGREDIENTS

- 1 teaspoon olive oil
- 1 1/2 cups water
- 1/2 cup chopped green bell pepper
- 1 tablespoon minced fresh basil
- 1/2 cup chopped onion
- 1 teaspoon chicken bouillon granules
- 1 clove garlic, minced
- 1/4 teaspoon ground black pepper
- 1 (14.5 ounce) can diced tomatoes
- 1 (10 ounce) package frozen chopped spinach, thawed

DIRECTIONS

1. In a large saucepan over medium heat, cook bell pepper, onion and garlic in oil until tender. Stir in tomatoes, water, basil, bouillon and black pepper. Bring to a boil, then reduce heat and simmer 10 minutes.
2. Stir in spinach and cook 5 to 7 minutes more.

VEGETABLE MEDLEY
Servings: 4 | Prep: 20m | Cooks: 15m | Total: 35m

NUTRITION FACTS

Calories: 66 | Carbohydrates: 12.6g | Fat: 1.5g | Protein: 3.3g | Cholesterol: 0mg

INGREDIENTS

- cooking spray
- 2 cups fresh mushrooms, sliced
- 1 tomato, diced
- 2 yellow squash, cubed

- 1 pinch garlic pepper seasoning
- 2 zucchini, cubed

DIRECTIONS

1. Spray a large skillet with cooking spray and add tomatoes. Cook over medium heat for 5 minutes and add garlic pepper. Stir in mushrooms, squash, and zucchini. Simmer until vegetables are tender-crisp, 10 to 15 minutes.

MEXICAN PINTO BEANS

Servings: 12 | Prep: 15m | Cooks: 2h45m | Total: 4h | Additional: 1h

NUTRITION FACTS

Calories: 159 | Carbohydrates: 23g | Fat: 3.2g | Protein: 10.2g | Cholesterol: 10.2mg

INGREDIENTS

- 1 pound dry pinto beans
- 1/2 pound bacon
- 4 serrano peppers

DIRECTIONS

1. Place the beans in a large pot with enough water to cover by 3 to 4 inches, and bring to a boil. Remove from heat, and let sit 1 hour. Drain water. Pour in enough fresh water to cover beans by 3 to 4 inches, and bring to a boil. Reduce heat, cover, and simmer 1 hour.
2. Place bacon in a skillet, and cook over medium high heat until evenly brown. Crumble bacon, and transfer, along with grease, to the pot with the beans. Continue to cook beans on low heat for 30 minutes.
3. Place the whole chile peppers into the pot, and continue cooking beans 1 hour, or until tender.

PUMPKIN SPICE COOKIES

Servings: 56 | Prep: 15m | Cooks: 25m | Total: 28m | Additional: 1m

NUTRITION FACTS

Calories: 74 | Carbohydrates: 12.6g | Fat: 2.2g | Protein: 1.4g | Cholesterol: 8mg

INGREDIENTS

- 2 1/2 cups all-purpose flour
- 2 tablespoons butter
- 1 cup rolled oats
- 1 1/3 cups light brown sugar

- 4 teaspoons baking powder
- 2 eggs
- 1 1/2 teaspoons ground cinnamon
- 1 teaspoon vanilla extract
- 1/2 teaspoon ground nutmeg
- 1 (15 ounce) can pumpkin
- 1 teaspoon pumpkin pie spice
- 1/2 cup apple butter
- 1/2 teaspoon ground ginger
- 1 cup chopped walnuts
- 1/4 teaspoon salt

DIRECTIONS

1. Preheat an oven to 375 degrees F (190 degrees C). Grease 2 baking sheets.
2. Stir the flour, oats, baking powder, cinnamon, nutmeg, pumpkin pie spice, ginger, and salt in a bowl.
3. Beat the butter and brown sugar with an electric mixer in a large bowl until smooth. Add 1 egg and allow it to blend into the mixture before adding the other along with the vanilla. Add the pumpkin and apple butter; continue beating. Mix in the flour mixture until just incorporated. Fold in the walnuts, mixing just enough to evenly combine. Drop spoonfuls of the dough 2 inches apart onto the prepared baking sheets.
4. Bake in the preheated oven until the edges are golden, about 12 minutes. Allow the cookies to cool on the baking sheet for 1 minute before removing to a wire rack to cool completely.

JORGE'S INDIAN-SPICED TOMATO LENTIL SOUP

Servings: 5 | Prep: 15m | Cooks: 20m | Total: 35m

NUTRITION FACTS

Calories: 179 | Carbohydrates: 32.5g | Fat: 1g | Protein: 11.1g | Cholesterol: 2mg

INGREDIENTS

- 4 cups low-sodium vegetable broth, divided
- 1/8 teaspoon garam masala
- 1 small yellow onion, finely chopped
- 1/8 teaspoon cayenne pepper
- 1 clove garlic, finely chopped
- 1 cup red lentils
- 1 teaspoon ground coriander
- 1 (14.5 ounce) can no-salt-added diced tomatoes, undrained
- 1/2 teaspoon ground cinnamon

- 1 tablespoon fresh lemon juice (optional)
- 1/8 teaspoon ground turmeric
- 1 tablespoon crumbled feta cheese (optional)

DIRECTIONS

1. Bring 1/2 cup broth to a boil in a pot; reduce heat and simmer. Add onion and garlic and simmer until onion is translucent and tender, about 5 minutes. Stir coriander, cinnamon, turmeric, garam masala, and cayenne pepper into onion mixture; simmer for 1 minute.
2. Stir lentils into spiced onion mixture; cook, stirring constantly, for 30 seconds. Add remaining 3 1/2 cups broth and tomatoes; bring to a boil. Reduce heat to low, cover, and simmer until lentils are tender, 10 to 12 minutes. Stir lemon juice into soup and garnish with feta cheese.

APPLESAUCE FOR THE FREEZER
Servings: 20 | Prep: 15m | Cooks: 25m | Total: 40m

NUTRITION FACTS

Calories: 63 | Carbohydrates: 16.6g | Fat: 0.1g | Protein: 0.2g | Cholesterol: 0mg

INGREDIENTS

- 3 1/2 pounds apples - peeled, cored, and quartered
- 3 tablespoons lemon juice, or more to taste
- 1 cup water
- 1 (3 inch) piece cinnamon stick
- 1/4 cup dark brown sugar
- 4 strips lemon zest
- 1/4 cup white sugar, or less to taste
- 1/2 teaspoon salt

DIRECTIONS

1. Stir apples, water, brown sugar, white sugar, lemon juice, cinnamon stick, lemon zest, and salt together in a large pot. Place a cover on the pot and bring the mixture to a boil. Reduce heat to medium-low and cook until the apples are soft, 20 to 30 minutes.
2. Remove pot from heat. Remove and discard cinnamon stick and lemon zest strips. Mash apples with a potato masher.

STIR-FRIED SNOW PEAS AND CARROTS
Servings: 2 | Prep: 10m | Cooks: 15m | Total: 25m

NUTRITION FACTS

Calories: 94 | Carbohydrates: 13.4g | Fat: 3g | Protein: 3.9g | Cholesterol: 2mg

INGREDIENTS

- 1 teaspoon soy sauce
- 1/2 pound snow peas
- 1 teaspoon cornstarch
- 1/2 cup thinly sliced carrot
- cooking spray
- 1/2 cup chicken broth
- 1 teaspoon sesame oil
- 1 teaspoon ground cumin

DIRECTIONS

1. Whisk together the soy sauce and cornstarch in a bowl until cornstarch is completely dissolved; set aside.
2. Prepare a skillet with cooking spray and place over medium heat; drizzle in the sesame oil. Place the snow peas and carrots in the skillet; stir-fry for 2 minutes. Pour the broth over the vegetables. Bring to a boil, cover, and reduce heat to low; simmer until vegetables are slightly softened, about 5 minutes. Stir in the soy sauce mixture; continue to stir-fry until the sauce has thickened.

ASPARAGUS GUACAMOLE

Servings: 4 | Prep: 15m | Cooks: 1h | Total: 1h15m

NUTRITION FACTS

Calories: 35 | Carbohydrates: 7.4g | Fat: 0.2g | Protein: 3g | Cholesterol: 0mg

INGREDIENTS

- 24 spears fresh asparagus, trimmed and coarsely chopped
- 2 cloves garlic
- 1/2 cup salsa
- 4 green onions, sliced
- 1 tablespoon chopped cilantro

DIRECTIONS

1. Place the asparagus in a pot with enough water to cover. Bring to a boil, and cook 5 minutes, until tender but firm. Drain, and rinse with cold water.
2. Place the asparagus, salsa, cilantro, garlic, and green onions in a food processor or blender, and process to desired consistency. Refrigerate 1 hour, or until chilled, before serving.

CABBAGE AND RICE

Servings: 8 | Prep: 15m | Cooks: 20m | Total: 35m

NUTRITION FACTS

Calories: 150 | Carbohydrates: 30.4g | Fat: 1.6g | Protein: 4.2g | Cholesterol: 0mg

INGREDIENTS

- 1 cup long grain white rice
- 1 clove garlic, crushed
- 2 cups water
- 1 head cabbage, cored and shredded
- 2 teaspoons olive oil
- 1 (14.5 ounce) can diced tomatoes
- 1 medium onion, chopped
- 1/2 cup jalapeno pepper rings

DIRECTIONS

1. In a saucepan, combine the rice and water. Bring to a boil. Cover and reduce heat to low. Simmer for 15 to 20 minutes, until water is absorbed and rice is tender.
2. Meanwhile, heat the olive oil in a large pot. Add the onion and garlic; cook and stir until fragrant, about 3 minutes. Add the cabbage, and cook for about 10 minutes, stirring occasionally, until the cabbage cooks down. Mix in the tomatoes, pepper rings and cooked rice. Simmer for 10 to 15 minutes to blend the flavors together.

GARBANZO BEAN BURGERS

Servings: 4 | Prep: 30m | Cooks: 30m | Total: 1h30m

NUTRITION FACTS

Calories: 140 | Carbohydrates: 21.7g | Fat: 4.2g | Protein: 4.9g | Cholesterol: 0mg

INGREDIENTS

- 1 (15 ounce) can garbanzo beans, rinsed and drained
- 2 tablespoons chopped fresh cilantro
- 1 red bell pepper, finely chopped
- 1 tablespoon tahini paste
- 1 carrot, grated
- salt and black pepper to taste
- 3 cloves garlic, minced
- 1 teaspoon olive oil (optional)

- 1 red chile pepper, seeded and minced

DIRECTIONS

1. Place garbanzo beans in the bowl of a food processor with bell pepper, carrot, garlic, red chile pepper, cilantro, tahini, salt, and pepper. Place the lid on the food processor, and pulse 5 times, then scrape the sides, and pulse the mixture until it is evenly mixed. If the mixture looks dry, add olive oil.
2. Refrigerate garbanzo bean burger mixture for 30 minutes.
3. Preheat an oven to 350 degrees F (175 degrees C). Prepare a baking sheet with parchment paper or lightly grease with cooking spray.
4. Shape the chilled garbanzo bean burger mixture into patties.
5. Bake 20 minutes, then carefully flip burgers and bake 10 more minutes, or until evenly browned.

GREEN BEANS AND POTATOES
Servings: 6 | Prep: 10m | Cooks: 25m | Total: 35m

NUTRITION FACTS

Calories: 83 | Carbohydrates: 18.3g | Fat: 0.2g | Protein: 2.1g | Cholesterol: 0mg

INGREDIENTS

- 3 cups thinly sliced potatoes
- 1 teaspoon vegetarian Worcestershire sauce
- 2 cups frozen green beans
- 1 cup vegetable broth, divided
- 1/2 teaspoon dried thyme
- 1 teaspoon cornstarch
- 1/4 teaspoon ground black pepper
- 1/4 cup chopped fresh parsley

DIRECTIONS

1. In a large skillet over medium-high heat combine potatoes, green beans, thyme, pepper, Worcestershire sauce and 3/4 cup of broth. Bring to a boil; reduce heat to medium-low, cover and simmer 15 to 20 minutes or until vegetables are tender.
2. In a small bowl blend remaining broth and cornstarch. Stir in parsley; add to potato mixture. Cook, stirring, until bubbly and thickened.

APPLE RAISIN CAKES
Servings: 6 | Prep: 10m | Cooks: 7m | Total: 17m

NUTRITION FACTS

Calories: 203 | Carbohydrates: 41.1g | Fat: 2.1g | Protein: 6.1g | Cholesterol: 62mg

INGREDIENTS

- 2 eggs, beaten
- 1/2 cup whole wheat flour
- 1 cup applesauce
- 2 teaspoons baking powder
- 1 teaspoon ground cinnamon
- 2 teaspoons vanilla extract
- 2 teaspoons white sugar
- 1/2 cup raisins
- 1 cup all-purpose flour

DIRECTIONS

1. In a large mixing bowl, combine eggs, applesauce, cinnamon, sugar, flour, baking powder, vanilla, and raisins. Form small cakes out of the batter.
2. Heat a nonstick griddle over medium heat, fry the cakes until both sides are browned, about 5 to 7 minutes.

FRUIT LEATHER

Servings: 16 | Prep: 20m | Cooks: 5h | Total: 5h20m

NUTRITION FACTS

Calories: 90 | Carbohydrates: 23.5g | Fat: 0.1g | Protein: 0.3g | Cholesterol: 0mg

INGREDIENTS

- 1 cup sugar
- 4 cups peeled, cored and chopped apple
- 1/4 cup lemon juice
- 4 cups peeled, cored and chopped pears

DIRECTIONS

1. Preheat the oven to 150 degrees F (65 degrees C). Cover a baking sheet with a layer of plastic wrap or parchment paper.
2. In the container of a blender, combine the sugar, lemon juice, apple and pear. Cover and puree until smooth. Spread evenly on the prepared pan. Place the pan on the top rack of the oven.
3. Bake for 5 to 6 hours, leaving the door to the oven partway open. Fruit is dry when the surface is no longer tacky and you can tear it like leather. Roll up on the plastic wrap and store in an airtight jar.

SPICY PASTA

Servings: 6 | Prep: 10m | Cooks: 20m | Total: 30m

NUTRITION FACTS

Calories: 134 | Carbohydrates: 22.5g | Fat: 2.8g | Protein: 4.4g | Cholesterol: 0mg

INGREDIENTS

- 1 (12 ounce) package rotini pasta
- 1 onion, diced
- 1 tablespoon vegetable oil
- 2 red chile peppers, seeded and chopped
- 1 clove garlic, crushed
- 1 (14.5 ounce) can diced tomatoes
- 1 teaspoon dried basil
- 3 drops hot pepper sauce
- 1 teaspoon Italian seasoning
- salt and ground black pepper to taste

DIRECTIONS

1. Bring a large pot of lightly salted water to a boil. Cook pasta in boiling water for 8 to 10 minutes, or until al dente; drain.
2. Meanwhile, heat oil in a saucepan over medium heat. Saute garlic with basil and Italian seasoning for 2 to 3 minutes. Stir in onion and chiles; cook until onion is tender. Stir in tomatoes and hot sauce; simmer for 5 minutes, or until heated through. Toss with the cooked pasta, and season with salt and pepper.

THANKSGIVING SPINACH SALAD

Servings: 4 | Prep: 10m | Cooks: 20m | Total: 30m

NUTRITION FACTS

Calories: 115 | Carbohydrates: 30g | Fat: 0.3g | Protein: 1.5g | Cholesterol: 0mg

INGREDIENTS

- 3/4 cup sweetened dried cranberries, chopped
- 2 teaspoons honey
- 1 McIntosh apple - peeled, cored, and diced
- 1 teaspoon chili powder
- 1/2 small red onion, finely chopped
- 1/2 teaspoon ground cinnamon

- 2 tablespoons lemon juice
- 1 (6 ounce) bag baby spinach, torn into bite-sized pieces

DIRECTIONS

1. Mix cranberries, apple, onion, lemon juice, honey, chili powder, and cinnamon together in a large bowl. Let rest for flavors to blend, about 20 minutes. Add spinach and toss to coat.

RUTABAGA OVEN FRIES

Servings: 4 | Prep: 10m | Cooks: 30m | Total: 40m

NUTRITION FACTS

Calories: 50 | Carbohydrates: 8.7g | Fat: 1.4g | Protein: 1.3g | Cholesterol: 0mg

INGREDIENTS

- 1 rutabaga, peeled and cut into spears
- 3 cloves garlic, minced
- 1 teaspoon olive oil
- 1 pinch salt to taste
- 4 sprigs fresh rosemary, minced

DIRECTIONS

1. Preheat oven to 400 degrees F (200 degrees C).
2. Combine rutabaga spears with oil, minced rosemary, garlic, and salt. Toss until evenly coated.
3. Lay rutabaga spears onto a baking sheet, leaving space between for even crisping. Bake until rutabaga fries are cooked through and crisped on the outside, about 30 minutes.

CLASSIC TURKEY AND RICE SOUP

Servings: 6 | Prep: 20m | Cooks: 25m | Total: 45m

NUTRITION FACTS

Calories: 115 | Carbohydrates: 22.4g | Fat: 1.7g | Protein: 3.2g | Cholesterol: 4mg

INGREDIENTS

- 1 turkey carcass
- water to cover
- 1 large onion, halved and skin left on
- 2 large onions, diced
- 1 large carrot, roughly chopped
- 2 carrots, diced

- 1 stalk celery, roughly chopped
- 2 stalks celery, diced
- 1 head garlic, halved
- 2 cloves garlic, minced
- 1 teaspoon dried rosemary
- 1 teaspoon poultry seasoning
- 1 teaspoon dried thyme
- 1 teaspoon dried rosemary
- 2 bay leaves
- 1 teaspoon onion powder
- salt and ground black pepper to taste
- 2 cups cooked rice

DIRECTIONS

1. Combine turkey carcass, halved onion, roughly chopped carrot, roughly chopped celery, halved garlic head, 1 teaspoon rosemary, thyme, bay leaves, salt, and pepper in a stockpot; pour in enough water to cover. Bring mixture to a boil, cover pot, reduce heat, and simmer until flavors have blended, about 1 hour.
2. Remove turkey carcass and pull remaining meat from bones; reserve meat and discard carcass. Remove vegetables and bay leaves from stock using a slotted spoon and discard.
3. Stir diced onions, diced carrots, diced celery, minced garlic, poultry seasoning, 1 teaspoon rosemary, and onion powder into stock; bring to a boil. Reduce heat, cover pot, and simmer until vegetables are very tender, 20 to 30 minutes. Add cooked rice and turkey meat to soup; season with salt and pepper. Cook until rice and turkey meat are warmed, about 5 minutes.

STIR-FRIED MUSHROOMS WITH BABY CORN
Servings: 4 | Prep: 10m | Cooks: 15m | Total: 25m

NUTRITION FACTS

Calories: 49 | Carbohydrates: 8.3g | Fat: 0.9g | Protein: 3.4g | Cholesterol: 0mg

INGREDIENTS

- 2 tablespoons cooking oil
- 1 tablespoon light soy sauce
- 3 cloves garlic, minced
- 1 tablespoon oyster sauce
- 1 onion, diced
- 2 teaspoons cornstarch
- 8 baby corn ears, sliced

- 3 tablespoons water
- 2/3 pound fresh mushrooms, sliced
- 1 red chile pepper, sliced
- 1 tablespoon fish sauce
- 1/4 cup chopped fresh cilantro

DIRECTIONS

1. Heat the oil in a large skillet or wok over medium heat; cook the garlic in the hot oil until browned, 5 to 7 minutes. Add the onion and baby corn and cook until the onion is translucent, 5 to 7 minutes. Add the mushrooms to the mixture and cook until slightly softened, about 2 minutes. Pour the fish sauce, soy sauce, and oyster sauce into the mixture and stir until incorporated.
2. Whisk the cornstarch and water together in a small bowl until the cornstarch is dissolved into the water; pour into the mushroom mixture. Cook and stir until thickened and glistening. Transfer to a serving dish; garnish with the chile pepper and cilantro to serve.

GOURMET MICROWAVE POPCORN
Servings: 2 | Prep: 5m | Cooks: 5m | Total: 10m

NUTRITION FACTS

Calories: 114 | Carbohydrates: 18.5g | Fat: 3.6g | Protein: 3g | Cholesterol: 0mg

INGREDIENTS

- 1/4 cup unpopped popcorn
- 1 teaspoon olive oil, or more if needed
- salt to taste

DIRECTIONS

1. Place popcorn in a brown paper bag. Tightly seal the bag by folding the top several times.
2. Microwave on High until the popping slows, about 2 minutes. Carefully open the bag. Season with salt and drizzle with olive oil. Reclose the bag and shake to distribute the seasoning.

MOROCCAN MASHED POTATOES
Servings: 6 | Prep: 20m | Cooks: 25m | Total: 45m

NUTRITION FACTS

Calories: 103 | Carbohydrates: 21.3g | Fat: 1.4g | Protein: 1.8g | Cholesterol: 0mg

INGREDIENTS

- 10 large baking potatoes, peeled and cubed

- 1 tablespoon salt, or to taste
- 3 tablespoons olive oil, or as needed
- 2 teaspoons ground black pepper
- 1 onion, diced
- 1/2 teaspoon ground cumin
- 1 tablespoon ground turmeric

DIRECTIONS

1. Place the potatoes into a large pot, and fill with enough water to cover. Bring to a boil over medium-high heat, and cook until tender and can be pierced with a fork, about 20 minutes.
2. Meanwhile, place 1 tablespoon olive oil in a skillet, and heat over medium-high heat. Stir in the onion and cook until translucent and lightly browned, about 6 minutes.
3. Drain water from the potatoes, and mash. Stir in the onion, and continue mashing. Mix in the turmeric, salt, pepper, and cumin. Add the remaining 2 tablespoons olive oil, or amount desired to make the potatoes more or less creamy.

BRUSSELS SPROUTS STIR FRY

Servings: 8 | Prep: 20m | Cooks: 15m | Total: 35m

NUTRITION FACTS

Calories: 86 | Carbohydrates: 15.5g | Fat: 2g | Protein: 3.2g | Cholesterol: 0mg

INGREDIENTS

- 1 tablespoon vegetable oil
- 1 red pepper, seeded and cut into 1/2-inch cubes
- 1 onion, chopped
- 1/4 cup chicken broth
- 1 large potato, peeled and cubed
- ground black pepper, to taste
- 1 bay leaf
- 2 tablespoons chopped green onions
- 1 pound Brussels sprouts, trimmed and halved

DIRECTIONS

1. Heat the vegetable oil in a skillet over medium heat. Stir in the onion, potato, and bay leaf. Cook and stir until the onion is transparent, about 5 minutes. Add the Brussels sprouts, red pepper, and chicken broth. Cover and cook until vegetables are tender, about 10 minutes. Remove the bay leaf. Toss with black pepper, to taste. Garnish with green onions, and serve immediately.

HERBED EGGPLANT SLICES

Servings: 4 | Prep: 15m | Cooks: 15m | Total: 30m

NUTRITION FACTS

Calories: 38 | Carbohydrates: 8.7g | Fat: 0.4g | Protein: 1.8g | Cholesterol: 0mg

INGREDIENTS

- 1 clove garlic, minced
- 1 eggplant, sliced into 1/2 inch rounds
- 1 tablespoon minced fresh oregano
- salt to taste
- 1/4 cup chopped fresh basil
- ground black pepper to taste
- 1/2 cup chopped fresh parsley

DIRECTIONS

1. Preheat oven to 400 degrees F (205 degrees C). Coat a baking sheet with cooking spray.
2. In a small bowl, combine garlic, oregano, basil ,and parsley. Mix well, and set aside.
3. Generously season each eggplant slice with salt and pepper on both sides. Place on baking sheet.
4. Bake 5 to 7 minutes on each side, until tender and slightly browned. Sprinkle herb mixture on eggplant slices, and place under the broiler for 30 seconds. Transfer to a serving plate, and serve immediately.

OVEN BAKED TEMPEH

Servings: 6 | Prep: 40m | Cooks: 30m | Total: 1h10m

NUTRITION FACTS

Calories: 118 | Carbohydrates: 13.8g | Fat: 2.8g | Protein: 7.7g | Cholesterol: 0mg

INGREDIENTS

- 1 1/2 teaspoons olive oil
- 2 cups baby carrots, halved
- 1/8 teaspoon crushed red pepper flakes
- 1 cup diced zucchini
- 1 leek, sliced
- 1 (8 ounce) package seasoned tempeh
- 1/3 cup shallots, chopped
- 1/2 cup dry sherry
- 1/2 cup red bell pepper, chopped
- 1 tomato, chopped

- 4 cloves garlic, minced
- 1 tablespoon tamari

DIRECTIONS

1. Preheat oven to 350 degrees F (175 degrees C).
2. Place oil and crushed red pepper in a stovetop-safe and oven proof 2 quart casserole dish. Saute over medium heat for 1 minute. Add leek, shallot, red bell pepper and garlic. Saute for 3 minutes. Add the carrots and zucchini. Saute, stirring frequently for 5 minutes. Add the tempeh and saute for 5 more minutes. Add the sherry, tomato and tamari. Saute for an additional 5 minutes.
3. Cover casserole dish and bake in at 350 degrees F (175 degrees C) for 30 minutes.

CURTIDO (EL SALVADORAN CABBAGE SALAD)
Servings: 4 | Prep: 20m | Cooks: 5m | Total: 45m

NUTRITION FACTS

Calories: 50 | Carbohydrates: 11.3g | Fat: 0.3g | Protein: 2.3g | Cholesterol: 0mg

INGREDIENTS

- 1/2 head green cabbage, cored and shredded
- 1 cup distilled white vinegar
- 1 carrot, grated
- 1/2 cup water
- 1 quart boiling water
- teaspoons dried oregano
- 3 green onions, minced

DIRECTIONS

1. Combine the cabbage and carrot in a large bowl and pour the boiling water over the mixture. Allow the mixture to steep for 5 minutes; drain well. Return the cabbage and carrots to the bowl. Mix in the green onion, vinegar, 1/2 cup of water, and oregano. Toss until all ingredients are combined. Chill for 20 minutes before serving.

SWEET POTATO HUMMUS
Servings: 20 | Prep: 20m | Cooks: 45m | Total: 1h20m

NUTRITION FACTS

Calories: 75 | Carbohydrates: 12.2g | Fat: 2.3g | Protein: 1.6g | Cholesterol: 0mg

INGREDIENTS

- 3 sweet potatoes
- 1/2 teaspoon lemon zest
- 1 (15 ounce) can garbanzo beans, drained (reserve liquid) and rinsed
- 1/4 teaspoon ground cumin
- 2 tablespoons extra-virgin olive oil
- 1/4 teaspoon ground coriander
- 2 tablespoons tahini
- 1/4 teaspoon ground white pepper
- 2 tablespoons lemon juice
- sea salt to taste

DIRECTIONS

1. Preheat oven to 400 degrees F (200 degrees C).
2. Poke holes all over sweet potatoes with a fork.
3. Roast sweet potatoes in the preheated oven until soft, about 45 minutes; let cool. Cut sweet potatoes in half lengthwise.
4. Combine garbanzo beans and olive oil in a blender and pulse several times to mash. Scoop flesh out of sweet potato peels and add to the blender; pulse to combine. Add tahini, lemon juice, lemon zest, cumin, coriander, white pepper, and sea salt to mixture; blend until smooth, adding reserved garbanzo bean liquid as needed to make a smooth, creamy hummus.

FRESH STRAWBERRY GRANITA
Servings: 8 | Prep: 10m | Cooks: 2h15 | Total: 2h25m

NUTRITION FACTS

Calories: 69 | Carbohydrates: 17.1g | Fat: 0.3g | Protein: 0.8g | Cholesterol: 0mg

INGREDIENTS

- 2 pounds ripe strawberries, hulled and halved
- 1/2 teaspoon lemon juice (optional)
- 1/3 cup white sugar, or to taste
- 1/4 teaspoon balsamic vinegar (optional)
- 1 cup water
- 1 tiny pinch salt

DIRECTIONS

1. Rinse strawberries with cold water; let drain. Transfer berries to a blender and add sugar, water, lemon juice, balsamic vinegar, and salt.

2. Pulse several times to get the mixture moving, then blend until smooth, about 1 minute. Pour into a large baking dish. Puree should only be about 3/8 inch deep in the dish.
3. Place dish uncovered in the freezer until mixture barely begins to freeze around the edges, about 45 minutes. Mixture will still be slushy in the center.
4. Lightly stir the crystals from the edge of the granita mixture into the center, using a fork, and mix thoroughly. Close freezer and chill until granita is nearly frozen, 30 to 40 more minutes. Mix lightly with a fork as before, scraping the crystals loose. Repeat freezing and stirring with the fork 3 to 4 times until the granita is light, crystals are separate, and granita looks dry and fluffy.
5. Portion granita into small serving bowls to serve.

OVEN BAKED TEMPEH

Servings: 6 | Prep: 20m | Cooks: 25m | Total: 45m

NUTRITION FACTS

Calories: 118 | Carbohydrates: 13.8g | Fat: 2.8g | Protein: 7.7g | Cholesterol: 0mg

INGREDIENTS

- 1 1/2 teaspoons olive oil
- 2 cups baby carrots, halved
- 1/8 teaspoon crushed red pepper flakes
- 1 cup diced zucchini
- 1 leek, sliced
- 1 (8 ounce) package seasoned tempeh
- 1/3 cup shallots, chopped
- 1/2 cup dry sherry
- 1/2 cup red bell pepper, chopped
- 1 tomato, chopped
- 4 cloves garlic, minced
- 1 tablespoon tamari

DIRECTIONS

1. Preheat oven to 350 degrees F (175 degrees C).
2. Place oil and crushed red pepper in a stovetop-safe and oven proof 2 quart casserole dish. Saute over medium heat for 1 minute. Add leek, shallot, red bell pepper and garlic. Saute for 3 minutes. Add the carrots and zucchini. Saute, stirring frequently for 5 minutes. Add the tempeh and saute for 5 more minutes. Add the sherry, tomato and tamari. Saute for an additional 5 minutes.
3. Cover casserole dish and bake in at 350 degrees F (175 degrees C) for 30 minutes.

EASY ROASTED POTATOES

Servings: 6 | Prep: 15m | Cooks: 40m | Total: 55m

NUTRITION FACTS

Calories: 128 | Carbohydrates: 24.6 g | Fat: 2.5g | Protein: 3g | Cholesterol: 0mg

INGREDIENTS

- 1 teaspoon McCormick® Dill Weed
- 1/4 teaspoon McCormick® Black Pepper, Coarse Ground
- 1 teaspoon McCormick® Garlic Powder
- 2 pounds red potatoes, cut into wedges
- 1/2 teaspoon salt
- 1 tablespoon olive oil

DIRECTIONS

1. Preheat oven to 400 degrees F. Mix dill weed, garlic powder, salt and pepper in small bowl. Set aside.
2. Toss potatoes with oil in large bowl. Sprinkle seasoning mixture over potatoes; toss to coat.
3. Spread potatoes in single layer on foil-lined 15x10x1-inch baking pan.
4. Bake 40 minutes or until potatoes are tender and golden brown.

POTATO SALAD

Servings: 4 | Prep: 40m | Cooks: 10m | Total: 50m

NUTRITION FACTS

Calories: 104 | Carbohydrates: 23.6g | Fat: 0.3g | Protein: 2.6g | Cholesterol: <1mg

INGREDIENTS

- 2 potatoes
- 1 stalk celery
- 2 tablespoons low-fat mayonnaise
- 1 green bell pepper, chopped
- 2 tablespoons fat free ranch dressing
- salt and pepper to taste
- 1/4 onion, chopped

DIRECTIONS

1. Bring a pot of salted water to boil, place potatoes in water. Boil until potatoes are tender. Drain well. Let the potatoes cool 30 minutes.
2. Peel the skin off of the potatoes and cube them.
3. In a medium size mixing bowl combine potatoes, mayonnaise, ranch dressing, onion, celery, green pepper, salt and pepper. Cover and refrigerate until well chilled.

SEAFOOD GUMBO STOCK

Servings: 8 | Prep: 15m | Cooks: 7h35m | Total: 7h50m

NUTRITION FACTS

Calories: 112 | Carbohydrates: 12.1g | Fat: 1.3g | Protein: 13.2g | Cholesterol: 86mg

INGREDIENTS

- shells from 1 pound shrimp
- 3 cloves garlic, sliced
- 5 quarts water
- 2 sprigs fresh parsley
- 4 carrots, sliced
- 5 whole cloves
- 4 onions, quartered
- 1 teaspoon ground black pepper
- 1/2 bunch celery, sliced
- 1 tablespoon dried basil
- 2 bay leaves
- 2 teaspoons dried thyme

DIRECTIONS

1. Bake shrimp shells at 375 degrees F (195 degrees C) until dried and starting to brown on edges.
2. In an 8-quart pot, combine water, carrots, onions, celery, bay leaves, garlic, parsley, cloves, pepper, basil, thyme and shrimp shells. Bring slowly to a boil.
3. Reduce heat, and cook 5 to 7 hours. Replace water as needed, 2 or 3 times, by pouring more water down the inside of the pot.
4. Remove stock from heat, and strain. Press all liquid from the shells and vegetables, then discard them. Return liquid to heat, and reduce to 2 to 3 quarts, or to taste.

FISH SINIGANG (TILAPIA) - FILIPINO SOUR BROTH DISH

Servings: 4 | Prep: 5m | Cooks: 10m | Total: 15m

NUTRITION FACTS

Calories: 112 | Carbohydrates: 13.4g | Fat: 1g | Protein: 13.1g | Cholesterol: 21mg

INGREDIENTS

- 1/2 pound tilapia fillets, cut into chunks
- 1/4 cup tamarind paste
- 1 small head bok choy, chopped
- 3 cups water

- 2 medium tomatoes, cut into chunks
- 2 dried red chile peppers (optional)
- 1 cup thinly sliced daikon radish

DIRECTIONS

1. In a medium pot, combine the tilapia, bok choy, tomatoes and radish. Stir together the tamarind paste and water; pour into the pot. Toss in the chili peppers if using. Bring to a boil, and cook for 5 minutes, or just until the fish is cooked through. Even frozen fish will cook in less than 10 minutes. Do not over cook or else the fish will fall apart. Ladle into bowls to serve.

MICROWAVE CORN-ON-THE-COB IN THE HUSK

Servings: 1 | Prep: 5m | Cooks: 5m | Total: 10m

NUTRITION FACTS

Calories: 77 | Carbohydrates: 17.1g | Fat: 1.1g | Protein: 2.9g | Cholesterol: 0mg

INGREDIENTS

- 1 ear fresh corn in the husk

DIRECTIONS

1. Rinse entire ear of corn under water briefly. Wrap corn in a paper towel and place on a microwave-safe plate.
2. Cook corn in the microwave oven until hot and cooked through, 3 to 5 minutes. Remove from microwave and let rest for 2 minutes. Remove corn husk.

OVEN FRIED OKRA

Servings: 4 | Prep: 10m | Cooks: 25m | Total: 35m

NUTRITION FACTS

Calories: 95 | Carbohydrates: 19.1g | Fat: 2g | Protein: 3.3g | Cholesterol: 0mg

INGREDIENTS

- 1 (16 ounce) package frozen cut okra
- 1/4 cup panko bread crumbs
- butter flavored cooking spray
- 1/2 teaspoon garlic salt
- 1/4 cup yellow cornmeal
- 1/4 teaspoon ground black pepper (optional)

DIRECTIONS

1. Preheat an oven to 375 degrees F (190 degrees C). Place a baking rack on top of a baking sheet or sheet pan.
2. Cook the frozen okra in the microwave using your microwave's frozen vegetable setting, or on high for 8 minutes. Drain and cool on paper towels, about 5 to 10 minutes. Spray generously with butter flavored cooking spray. Add the cornmeal, panko bread crumbs, garlic salt, and pepper to a plastic food storage bag. Place the okra into the bag and shake to coat the okra with the cornmeal mixture.
3. Remove the okra from the bag and spread it on the prepared baking rack. Bake in the preheated oven until golden brown and crispy, about 15 to 20 minutes.

GRILLED ASIAN ASPARAGUS
Servings: 5 | Prep: 5m | Cooks: 5m | Total: 40m

NUTRITION FACTS

Calories: 84 | Carbohydrates: 15.1g | Fat: 1.9g | Protein: 3.2g | Cholesterol: 0mg

INGREDIENTS

- 1 pound fresh asparagus, trimmed
- sesame seeds
- 1/2 cup hoisin sauce

DIRECTIONS

1. Place asparagus and hoisin sauce into a resealable plastic bag and shake several times to coat asparagus with sauce. Allow to stand at least 30 minutes. For best flavor, refrigerate and marinate overnight.
2. Preheat an outdoor grill for medium heat and lightly oil the grate.
3. Remove asparagus from bag and shake off excess hoisin sauce; lay asparagus spears onto the grill and cook, turning every 1 to 2 minutes, until all sides of the spears show grill marks and hoisin sauce has caramelized onto the asparagus, 4 to 6 minutes.
4. Transfer asparagus to a serving platter and sprinkle with sesame seeds to serve.

SAUTEED KALE WITH APPLES
Servings: 4 | Prep: 15m | Cooks: 15m | Total: 30m

NUTRITION FACTS

Calories: 123 | Carbohydrates: 21.6g | Fat: 4g | Protein: 3g | Cholesterol: 0mg

INGREDIENTS

- 1 tablespoon olive oil
- 1/8 teaspoon sea salt

- 1 white onion, sliced
- 1/8 teaspoon ground black pepper
- 2 Red Delicious apples, cored and cut into bite-size pieces
- 4 cups chopped kale leaves
- 2 teaspoons apple cider vinegar

DIRECTIONS

1. Heat olive oil in a large skillet over medium heat; cook and stir onion until tender, about 4 minutes. Add apples, vinegar, salt, and pepper; cover skillet and cook until apples are tender, about 3 minutes. Add kale; cover and cook until kale is tender, 4 to 5 minutes.

ZUCCHINI-TOMATO SAUTE

Servings: 15 | Prep: 20m | Cooks: 1h | Total: 1h20m

NUTRITION FACTS

Calories: 92 | Carbohydrates: 9.9g | Fat: 1g | Protein: 13.2g | Cholesterol: 22mg

INGREDIENTS

- 8 tilapia fillets
- 1 large red onion, finely diced
- 15 limes, juiced
- 2 cucumbers, peeled, seeded, and finely diced
- 1 large tomato, finely diced
- 1/2 bunch finely chopped cilantro
- salt and pepper to taste

DIRECTIONS

1. Chop the raw tilapia into small pieces, and place in a large bowl. Pour in enough lime juice to cover the fish.
2. Mix the tomato, red onion, and cucumbers into the bowl. Stir in the cilantro. Season with salt and pepper.
3. Allow the ceviche to marinate, refrigerated, for at least an hour. Taste for seasoning before serving; add salt and pepper if necessary.

CHICKEN GUMBO SOUP

Servings: 8 | Prep: 10m | Cooks: 3h20m | Total: 3h30m

NUTRITION FACTS

Calories: 116 | Carbohydrates: 20.5g | Fat: 0.7g | Protein: 7.5g | Cholesterol: 9mg

INGREDIENTS

- 8 cups water
- 1/4 cup uncooked wild rice
- 1 teaspoon garlic powder
- 1 skinless, boneless chicken breast half - cut into cubes
- 1 tablespoon hot pepper sauce
- 1 1/2 cups uncooked rotini pasta
- 2 carrots, sliced thin
- salt to taste
- 4 ounces fresh mushrooms
- ground black pepper to taste
- 1 (10 ounce) package frozen okra, thawed and sliced
- 3 green onions, thinly sliced

DIRECTIONS

1. Bring the water to a boil. Add the garlic powder and the hot pepper sauce. Put the carrots and mushrooms into the pot of water. Cook for five minutes.
2. Add the okra, wild rice, and chicken cubes. Turn heat to low, and cook for three hours.
3. Add the spiral pasta, and cook for ten minutes. Add salt and pepper to taste. Serve hot, garnished with green onions.

CHLOE'S QUICK FRUIT SALAD
Servings: 4 | Prep: 15m | Cooks: 30m | Total: 45m

NUTRITION FACTS

Calories: 90 | Carbohydrates: 20.6g | Fat: 0.7g | Protein: 2.3g | Cholesterol: 1mg

INGREDIENTS

- 1 apple, cored and chopped
- 1 nectarine, pitted and chopped
- 1 large orange, peeled, sectioned, and cut into bite-size
- 1/4 cup fresh orange juice
- 1/2 cup seedless grapes
- 6 tablespoons plain low-fat yogurt

DIRECTIONS

1. In a mixing bowl, combine the apple, orange, grapes and nectarine. If using a passion fruit, spoon out the flesh and chop.
2. Pour enough fresh juice to coat and prevent oxidation. Toss and refrigerate.
3. Serve with dollop of low-fat yogurt.

MANHATTAN CLAM CHOWDER
Servings: 8 | Prep: 20m | Cooks: 25m | Total: 45m

NUTRITION FACTS

Calories: 82 | Carbohydrates: 15.8g | Fat: 0.2g | Protein: 3.9g | Cholesterol: 5mg

INGREDIENTS

- 1 pint shucked clams
- 1/4 cup chopped green onions
- 1 cup tomato and clam juice cocktail
- 1/4 teaspoon ground black pepper
- 2 potatoes, cleaned and chopped
- 1 (14.5 ounce) can Italian-style diced tomatoes
- 1 cup chopped green bell pepper

DIRECTIONS

1. Chop clams, reserving juice; set clams aside. Strain clam juice to remove bits of shell. Measure juice; add enough water to equal 1 1/2 cups liquid.
2. Combine clam juice mixture, clam-tomato juice cocktail, potatoes, bell peppers, scallions and black pepper in large saucepan; heat to a boil. Reduce heat; cover and simmer for about 15 minutes or until potatoes are just tender.
3. Stir in the undrained tomatoes and the chopped clams and heat through.

BANGAN KA BHURTA (INDIAN EGGPLANT)
Servings: 4 | Prep: 15m | Cooks: 15m | Total: 35m

NUTRITION FACTS

Calories: 61 | Carbohydrates: 11.8g | Fat: 1.5g | Protein: 2g | Cholesterol: 0mg

INGREDIENTS

- 1 eggplant
- 1/4 teaspoon ground cayenne pepper
- 1 teaspoon vegetable oil
- 1/4 teaspoon salt
- 1 medium onion, chopped

- 1/4 teaspoon pepper
- 2 roma (plum) tomatoes, chopped
- 4 sprigs chopped fresh cilantro

DIRECTIONS

1. Preheat the oven broiler. Place eggplant in a roasting pan, and broil 5 minutes, turning occasionally, until about 1/2 the skin is scorched.
2. Place eggplant in microwave safe dish. Cook 5 minutes on High in the microwave, or until tender. Cool enough to handle, and remove skin, leaving some scorched bits. Cut into thick slices.
3. Heat oil in a skillet over medium heat, stir in the onion, and cook until tender. Mix in eggplant, and tomatoes. Season with cayenne pepper, salt, and black pepper. Continue to cook and stir until soft. Garnish with cilantro to serve.

MEXICAN HOT CARROTS

Servings: 8 | Prep: 15m | Cooks: 15m | Total: 8h30m

NUTRITION FACTS

Calories: 45 | Carbohydrates: 10.5g | Fat: 0.2g | Protein: 1.1g | Cholesterol: 0mg

INGREDIENTS

- 6 carrots, peeled and sliced
- 1 (16 ounce) jar sliced jalapeno peppers, with liquid
- 2 onions, thinly sliced
- 1 cup vinegar

DIRECTIONS

1. Place the carrots in a saucepan with enough water to cover and cook over medium heat until nearly boiling, 7 to 10 minutes. Immediately drain the carrots and set aside to cool.
2. Divide the cooled carrots into two 1-quart glass jars. Alternate layers of onion and jalapeno peppers atop the carrots until the jars are full.
3. Mix the liquid from the jalapeno peppers and the vinegar in a saucepan; bring the mixture to a rolling boil. Remove from heat and pour the liquid into the jars until full. Seal the jars with lids. Place the jars in the refrigerator until cold, at least 8 hours.

ITALIAN ROASTED CAULIFLOWER

Servings: 4 | Prep: 25m | Cooks: 30m | Total: 1h55m

NUTRITION FACTS

Calories: 90 | Carbohydrates: 14.7g | Fat: 2.7g | Protein: 3.7g | Cholesterol: 0mg

INGREDIENTS

- 1 head cauliflower, cut into florets
- 3 tablespoons balsamic vinegar
- 1 large red bell pepper, cut into 1-1/2 inch pieces
- 2 tablespoons white wine vinegar
- 1 red onion, sliced
- 2 teaspoons olive oil
- 1/2 cup chopped fresh dill
- salt and pepper to taste

DIRECTIONS

1. Combine the cauliflower, bell pepper, onion, dill, balsamic vinegar, white wine vinegar, and olive oil in a large resalable bag; shake bag to evenly coat. Allow to marinate in refrigerator 1 to 2 hours, turning bag occasionally.
2. Preheat oven to 450 degrees F (230 degrees C).
3. Open the bag and season with salt and pepper; reseal the bag and shake again to coat. Pour into a 9x13 glass baking dish.
4. Bake in the preheated oven until tender, about 30 minutes, stirring occasionally.

SQUASH AND GREEN BEAN SAUTE SIDE DISH

Servings: 2 | Prep: 15m | Cooks: 10m | Total: 25m

NUTRITION FACTS

Calories: 89 | Carbohydrates: 19.6g | Fat: 0.9g | Protein: 5.1g | Cholesterol: 0mg

INGREDIENTS

- 2 yellow squash, sliced
- 1 tablespoon dried parsley
- 1 1/2 cups green beans
- 1/2 teaspoon ground coriander
- 1 1/2 cups halved cherry tomatoes
- 1/8 teaspoon salt, or to taste
- 2 tablespoons fresh lemon juice
- 1/8 teaspoon ground black pepper, or to taste

DIRECTIONS

1. Cook and stir squash and green beans in a nonstick skillet over medium heat until slightly softened, 2 to 3 minutes. Stir tomatoes, lemon juice, parsley, coriander, salt, and black pepper into squash mixture; cook and stir until tomatoes have softened, 5 to 10 minutes.

CURRIED COTTAGE FRIES

Servings: 8 | Prep: 10m | Cooks: 20m | Total: 30m

NUTRITION FACTS

Calories: 162 | Carbohydrates: 28.5g | Fat: 4.1g | Protein: 3.8g | Cholesterol: <1mg

INGREDIENTS

- 6 potatoes, cut into wedges
- 1 teaspoon paprika
- 2 tablespoons vegetable oil
- 1 teaspoon salt
- 2 tablespoons shredded Parmesan cheese
- 1/2 teaspoon garlic powder
- 2 teaspoons curry powder

DIRECTIONS

4. Preheat oven to 400 degrees F (200 degrees C). Grease a baking sheet.

1. Place potatoes, vegetable oil, Parmesan cheese, curry powder, paprika, salt, and garlic powder in a resealable plastic bag; shake to coat. Spread seasoned potatoes over prepared baking sheet.
2. Bake in preheated oven until tender, about 20 minutes.

TOMATO AND ZUCCHINI MELANGE

Servings: 2 | Prep: 5m | Cooks: 5m | Total: 10m

NUTRITION FACTS

Calories: 47 | Carbohydrates: 10.2g | Fat: 0.6g | Protein: 3g | Cholesterol: 0mg

INGREDIENTS

- 2 plum tomatoes, halved and cut into 1/4 inch slices
- 1/2 teaspoon dried oregano
- 1 large zucchini, sliced
- 1/4 teaspoon dried basil
- 3 tablespoons salsa
- salt and pepper to taste
- 3 tablespoons water

DIRECTIONS

1. In a small saucepan, mix together tomatoes, zucchini, salsa, water, oregano, basil, salt, and pepper. Mix in bell peppers if desired. Bring to a boil over medium heat, then reduce to a simmer. Simmer 3 to 4 minutes, stirring frequently.

MILLET-STUFFED PEPPERS
Servings: 5 | Prep: 10m | Cooks: 25m | Total: 35m

NUTRITION FACTS

Calories: 189 | Carbohydrates: 37.6g | Fat: 2.1g | Protein: 6.1g | Cholesterol: 0mg

INGREDIENTS

- 1 cup millet
- 5 medium bell peppers
- 4 cups water
- 3 medium tomatoes, chopped
- 4 cubes vegetable bouillon
- 1 (15 ounce) can black beans, drained

DIRECTIONS

1. Combine the millet, water and vegetable bouillon in a saucepan, and bring to a boil. Reduce heat to low, cover, and simmer for 15 minutes, or until the water is absorbed.
2. Slice the tops off of the peppers, and remove the seeds and cores. Set aside. When the millet is done, stir in the tomatoes and black beans. Spoon into the peppers until filled. Place the peppers into a glass baking dish, and cover with plastic wrap.
3. Cook in the microwave for 10 minutes, or until peppers are tender. Turn peppers every 2 to 3 minutes to ensure even cooking.

SLOW COOKER CHOCOLATE BANANA STEEL CUT OATS
Servings: 12 | Prep: 5m | Cooks: 6h | Total: 6h5m

NUTRITION FACTS

Calories: 180 | Carbohydrates: 36.9g | Fat: 2.6g | Protein: 6g | Cholesterol: 0mg

INGREDIENTS

- cooking spray
- 2 pounds ripe bananas, mashed
- 10 cups water
- 1/2 cup unsweetened cocoa powder
- 2 cups steel-cut oats
- 1/3 cup granular no-calorie sucralose sweetener (such as Splenda®) (optional)

DIRECTIONS

1. Lightly spray a 5-quart or larger slow cooker crock with cooking spray.
2. Mix water, oats, mashed bananas, cocoa powder, and sweetener in prepared slow cooker.
3. Cook on Low for 6 hours.

FRIED YELLOW SQUASH

Servings: 4 | Prep: 10m | Cooks: 15m | Total: 25m

NUTRITION FACTS

Calories: 130 | Carbohydrates: 21.2g | Fat: 4g | Protein: 3g | Cholesterol: <1mg

INGREDIENTS

- 3/4 cup self-rising cornbread mix (such as Martha White®)
- 2 yellow squash, cut into 1/8-inch slices
- salt and ground black pepper to taste
- 1/4 cup olive oil, or more as needed

DIRECTIONS

1. Place cornbread mix in a gallon-size resealable bag; season with salt and black pepper. Add squash, seal bag, and shake to coat evenly. Remove squash from bag and shake off any excess cornmeal.
2. Heat about 1/4 inch of olive oil in a large skillet over medium heat. Fry squash in the hot oil, working in batches, until center is cooked and edges are crisp, 2 to 3 minutes per side. Remove with a slotted spoon and drain on a paper towel-lined plate.

PAT'S BAKED OATMEAL

Servings: 15 | Prep: 15m | Cooks: 25m | Total: 40m

NUTRITION FACTS

Calories: 224 | Carbohydrates: 39.7g | Fat: 4.3g | Protein: 7.7g | Cholesterol: 44mg

INGREDIENTS

- 6 cups rolled oats
- 1/4 cup flax seed meal (optional)
- 4 eggs, beaten
- 3 tablespoons wheat germ (optional)
- 2 cups frozen blueberries
- 1 tablespoon baking powder
- 1 cup applesauce

- 1 tablespoon ground cinnamon
- 1 cup brown sugar
- 2 teaspoons vanilla extract
- 2 cups skim milk
- 1/2 teaspoon salt

DIRECTIONS

1. Preheat oven to 350 degrees F (175 degrees C).
2. Mix oats, eggs, blueberries, applesauce, brown sugar, skim milk, flax seed meal, wheat germ, baking powder, cinnamon, vanilla, and salt together in a large bowl; pour into a 9x13-inch baking dish.
3. Bake in preheated oven until the moisture is absorbed and the oats are tender, 25 to 32 minutes.

SUGAR-FREE AND DAIRY-FREE SLOW COOKER STEEL-CUT OATMEAL

Servings: 6 | Prep: 10m | Cooks: 3h | Total: 3h10m

NUTRITION FACTS

Calories: 159 | Carbohydrates: 32.8g | Fat: 1.8g | Protein: 4g | Cholesterol: 0mg

INGREDIENTS

- 2 bananas, mashed
- 1/4 cup raisins (optional)
- 5 cups water, divided
- 1 teaspoon cinnamon
- 1 cup steel cut oats
- 1 teaspoon vanilla extract

DIRECTIONS

1. Put bananas into a blender with 1 cup water; puree and pour into a slow cooker. Add remaining water, oats, raisins, cinnamon, and vanilla extract.
2. Cook on Medium, stirring every 30 minutes, for 3 hours.

YELLOW SQUASH AND ZUCCHINI DELIGHT

Servings: 4 | Prep: 15m | Cooks: 25m | Total: 40m

NUTRITION FACTS

Calories: 63 | Carbohydrates: 12.3g | Fat: 0.3g | Protein: 4.8g | Cholesterol: 0mg

INGREDIENTS

- 1 zucchini, sliced
- 1 large onion, sliced
- 1 yellow squash, sliced
- 1 (14.5 ounce) can fat-free chicken broth
- 1/2 small head cabbage, sliced

DIRECTIONS

1. In a large pot place zucchini, yellow squash, cabbage and onion. Pour broth over vegetables and bring to a boil over medium heat. Reduce heat to low, cover and simmer for 20 to 30 minutes.

TABBOULEH

Servings: 11 | Prep: 20m | Cooks: 1h30m | Total: 1h50m

NUTRITION FACTS

Calories: 118 | Carbohydrates: 18.9g | Fat: 4.2g | Protein: 3.3g | Cholesterol: 0mg

INGREDIENTS

- 1 1/2 cups bulgur
- 1/4 cup minced fresh mint leaves
- 3 cups boiling water
- 3 tablespoons olive oil
- 2 pounds tomatoes, diced
- 1/4 cup fresh lemon juice
- 1 cup chopped fresh parsley
- salt to taste
- 3 green onions, minced
- ground black pepper to taste

DIRECTIONS

1. Place bulgur in a casserole dish, and cover it with 3 cups boiling water. Cover. Let stand 30 minutes, or until the water has been absorbed.
2. Fluff bulgur with a fork. Add tomatoes, parsley, green onions, mint, olive oil, lemon juice, salt and pepper; stir to combine. Cover, and refrigerate for 1 to 2 hours. Serve either chilled or at room temperature.

BANANA OAT AND BRAN COOKIES

Servings: 5 | Prep: 5m | Cooks: 10m | Total: 15m

NUTRITION FACTS

Calories: 117 | Carbohydrates: 27.6g | Fat: 0.5g | Protein: 2.7g | Cholesterol: 1mg

INGREDIENTS

- 2 ripe bananas, mashed
- 1/5 cup real maple syrup
- 1/2 cup whole wheat flour
- 2 egg whites
- 1/4 cup wheat bran
- 1 teaspoon ground cinnamon
- 1/4 cup rolled oats
- 1/2 teaspoon salt
- 1/2 cup packed brown sugar
- 1/2 teaspoon baking powder
- 1/2 cup low-fat plain yogurt
- 1/2 cup raisins

DIRECTIONS

1. Preheat oven to 350 degrees F (175 degrees C).
2. Beat mashed bannanas, egg whites, brown sugar, maple syrup, yogurt, and cinnamon.
3. Combine the remaining dry ingredients: flour, oats, wheat bran, salt and baking powder in a separate bowl. Use an electric mixer to combine dry ingredients with wet mixture.
4. Add in raisins, chopped prunes, and/ or nuts.
5. Roll cookies into balls, place on a cookie sheet coated with cooking spray. Bake for 8-12 minutes until cookies are firm and dry.

WARM CHICKEN AND MANGO SALAD
Servings: 4 | Prep: 15m | Cooks: 15m | Total: 30m

NUTRITION FACTS

Calories: 275 | Carbohydrates: 29.9g | Fat: 4.3g | Protein: 30.8g | Cholesterol: 69mg

INGREDIENTS

- 1/3 cup vanilla low-fat yogurt
- 1 teaspoon olive oil
- 1 1/2 tablespoons lime juice
- 4 skinless, boneless chicken breast halves - cut into strips
- 1 1/2 tablespoons mango chutney
- 2 teaspoons grated fresh ginger
- 1 tablespoon seasoned rice vinegar
- 1 clove garlic, peeled and minced

- 1 teaspoon honey
- 1 1/2 cups peeled, seeded and chopped mango
- 1/4 teaspoon ground cumin
- 1 cup sliced red bell pepper
- 1/4 teaspoon ground coriander
- 1/3 cup chopped green onion
- 1/4 teaspoon ground paprika
- 8 cups torn romaine lettuce

DIRECTIONS

1. In a small bowl, blend vanilla yogurt, lime juice, mango chutney, rice vinegar, honey, cumin, coriander, and paprika.
2. Heat olive oil in a medium skillet over medium heat. Place chicken, ginger, and garlic in the skillet. Cook 7 to 10 minutes, stirring occasionally, until chicken is no longer pink and juices run clear.
3. Mix mango, red bell pepper, and green onions into the skillet. Cook about 5 minutes, until pepper is tender and mangoes are heated through. Stir in the vanilla yogurt mixture. Spoon over romaine lettuce to serve.

FRIJOLES

Servings: 12 | Prep: 10m | Cooks: 5h | Total: 5h10m

NUTRITION FACTS

Calories: 156 | Carbohydrates: 24.9g | Fat: 2.6 g | Protein: 8.3g | Cholesterol: 2mg

INGREDIENTS

- 1 pound dried pinto beans, washed
- 3 cloves garlic, minced
- 1 white onion, chopped
- 2 tablespoons lard
- 1/2 bunch fresh cilantro, chopped
- water to cover
- 1 fresh jalapeno pepper, chopped
- salt to taste

DIRECTIONS

1. Place beans in a large pot with onion, cilantro, jalapeno pepper, garlic, and lard; add enough water to cover with 4 to 5 inches of water. Bring to a boil, reduce heat, and cook for 2 to 3 hours. Depending on the beans, it may take up to 5 hours. Add more water if necessary.
2. When beans are soft, season to taste with salt.

SECRET INGREDIENT PICO DE GALLO

Servings: 4 | Prep: 20m | Cooks: 1h | Total: 1h20m

NUTRITION FACTS

Calories: 49 | Carbohydrates: 10.9g | Fat: 0.5g | Protein: 2.2g | Cholesterol: 0mg

INGREDIENTS

- 1/2 cup minced onion
- 4 large tomatoes, seeded and diced
- 2 jalapeno peppers, seeded and minced
- 1 tablespoon fresh lime juice
- 1/4 cup diced red bell pepper
- 1/4 cup chopped cilantro
- 1/4 cup minced dill pickle
- salt and pepper to taste

DIRECTIONS

1. In a medium bowl, combine the onion, jalapeno pepper, bell pepper, dill pickle, and diced tomatoes. Stir in lime juice and cilantro; season to taste with salt and pepper. Cover, and refrigerate at least 1 hour before serving, preferably overnight.

CHICKEN SOUP WITH ADZUKI BEANS, ESCAROLE, AND SWEET POTATO

Servings: 12 | Prep: 15m | Cooks: 2h | Total: 2h15m

NUTRITION FACTS

Calories: 169 | Carbohydrates: 29.1g | Fat: 1.9g | Protein: 9.9g | Cholesterol: 14mg

INGREDIENTS

- 1 1/2 quarts chicken broth
- 1 tablespoon dried thyme
- 4 boneless, skinless chicken thighs
- 1 tablespoon dried rosemary
- 1 cup dry adzuki beans
- 1 large sweet potato, peeled and cubed
- 1 cup uncooked wild rice
- 1 zucchini, cubed
- 2 onions, cut into large chunks

- 1 yellow squash, cubed
- 1 tablespoon bottled minced garlic
- 1/3 medium head escarole, coarsely chopped
- 1 teaspoon dried sage

DIRECTIONS

1. Place the chicken broth in a large pot. Mix in the chicken thighs, adzuki beans, wild rice, onions, and garlic. Season with sage, thyme, and rosemary. Bring to a boil, reduce heat, and cook 1 hour.
2. Remove chicken from the pot, shred with a fork, and set aside.
3. Stir the sweet potato into the pot. Continue cooking about 5 minutes, until sweet potato is slightly tender. Mix in the zucchini, yellow squash, and escarole. Continue cooking 15 minutes.
4. Return the shredded chicken to the pot. Cook until heated through. Increase the amount of broth if the soup seems too thick.

SEASONED ROASTED ROOT VEGETABLES
Servings: 10 | Prep: 30m | Cooks: 45m | Total: 1h15m

NUTRITION FACTS

Calories: 149 | Carbohydrates: 29.9g | Fat: 3.1g | Protein: 3.4g | Cholesterol: 0mg

INGREDIENTS

- olive oil cooking spray
- 3 carrots, cut into large chunks
- 1 butternut squash - peeled, seeded, and cut into 1-inch pieces
- 2 tablespoons olive oil, or as needed
- 1 large sweet potato, peeled and cut into 1-inch cubes
- 1 teaspoon ground thyme
- 1 (10 ounce) package frozen Brussels sprouts, thawed and halved
- 1 teaspoon dried rosemary
- 1 onion, halved and thickly sliced
- 1 pinch salt
- 1 parsnip, peeled and sliced
- ground black pepper to taste

DIRECTIONS

1. Preheat oven to 400 degrees F (200 degrees C). Spray a baking sheet with cooking spray.
2. Combine butternut squash, sweet potato, Brussels sprouts, onion, parsnip, and carrots in a large bowl. Drizzle with olive oil and toss to coat. Add thyme, rosemary, salt, and black pepper; toss again. Transfer coated vegetables to the prepared baking sheet.
3. Roast vegetables in the preheated oven for 25 minutes; stir and continue roasting until vegetables are slightly brown and tender, about 20 more minutes.

WHAT THE ELLE...BAKED EGG ROLLS
Servings: 8 | Prep: 15m | Cooks: 20m | Total: 35m

NUTRITION FACTS

Calories: 150 | Carbohydrates: 16.9g | Fat: 3.6g | Protein: 12.4g | Cholesterol: 28mg

INGREDIENTS

- 2 cups grated carrots
- 1 tablespoon water
- 1 (14.5 ounce) can bean sprouts, drained
- 1 tablespoon light soy sauce
- 1/2 cup chopped water chestnuts
- 1 teaspoon vegetable oil
- 1/4 cup chopped green bell pepper
- 1 teaspoon brown sugar
- 1/4 cup chopped green onions
- 1 pinch cayenne pepper
- 1 clove garlic, minced
- 16 egg roll wrappers
- 2 cups finely diced cooked chicken
- nonstick cooking spray
- 4 teaspoons cornstarch

DIRECTIONS

1. Preheat oven to 425 degrees F (220 degrees C). Lightly grease a baking sheet.
2. Coat a large skillet with nonstick cooking spray and heat over medium heat; cook and stir carrots, bean sprouts, water chestnuts, green pepper, green onions, and garlic until vegetables are crisp, about 3 minutes. Stir in chicken until heated through, 3 to 5 minutes.
3. Combine cornstarch, water, soy sauce, 1 teaspoon oil, brown sugar, and cayenne in a small bowl; stir into chicken mixture. Bring to a boil over high heat and stir, cooking until sauce is thickened, about 2 minutes; remove from heat.
4. Spoon 1/4 cup chicken mixture on the bottom third of one egg roll wrapper. Fold sides toward center and roll tightly; place seam side down on prepared baking sheet. Repeat with remaining filling and wrappers. Spray top of egg rolls with nonstick cooking spray.
5. Bake in preheated oven until lightly browned, 10 to 15 minutes.

EASY BAKED APPLES
Servings: 6 | Prep: 5m | Cooks: 1h | Total: 1h5m

NUTRITION FACTS

Calories: 55 | Carbohydrates: 14.6g | Fat: 0.2g | Protein: 0.4g | Cholesterol: 0mg

INGREDIENTS

- 6 small apples, cored and halved
- 2 cups sugar-free diet orange-flavored carbonated beverage

DIRECTIONS

1. Preheat an oven to 350 degrees F (175 degrees C).
2. Arrange the apples into a baking dish with the cut sides facing down. Pour the orange beverage over the apples.
3. Bake in the preheated oven until the apples are tender, about 1 hour.

REFRESHING SWEET AND SPICY JICAMA SALAD (VEGAN)

Servings: 6 | Prep: 20m | Cooks: 30m | Total: 50m

NUTRITION FACTS

Calories: 119 | Carbohydrates: 28.3g | Fat: 0.5g | Protein: 3.3g | Cholesterol: 0mg

INGREDIENTS

- 1 large jicama, peeled and julienned
- 4 radishes, thinly sliced
- 2 navel oranges, peeled and cut into chunks
- 3 Thai chile peppers, minced
- 1 large red bell pepper, cut into bite-size pieces
- 1/2 jalapeno pepper, diced
- 1/2 hothouse cucumber, diced
- 1/2 bunch cilantro, chopped
- 3 small sweet yellow peppers, sliced
- 1 lemon, juiced
- 2 small sweet orange peppers, sliced
- ground black pepper to taste

DIRECTIONS

1. Combine jicama, orange chunks, red bell pepper, cucumber, sweet yellow and orange peppers, radishes, Thai chile peppers, jalapeno pepper, cilantro, lemon juice, and black pepper in a large bowl.
2. Cover the bowl with plastic wrap and refrigerate until flavors blend, about 30 minutes.

TUNA-STUFFED ZUCCHINI

Servings: 6 | Prep: 25m | Cooks: 25m | Total: 50m

NUTRITION FACTS

Calories: 193 | Carbohydrates: 18.2g | Fat: 4.7g | Protein: 19.4g | Cholesterol: 48mg

INGREDIENTS

- 3 zucchini, ends trimmed
- 1 cup dry bread crumbs
- 4 (3 ounce) cans tuna, drained and flaked
- 1 egg, beaten
- 1/4 onion, grated
- salt and ground black pepper to taste
- 1 tomato, finely chopped (optional)
- 1 tablespoon olive oil

DIRECTIONS

1. Fill a large pot with salted water, place the zucchini into the pot, and boil over medium heat for about 5 minutes to soften. Remove the zucchini, slice in half lengthwise, and allow to cool.
2. Preheat oven to 350 degrees F (175 degrees C). Lightly grease a 9x13-inch baking dish.
3. Scoop out the flesh from the zucchini halves, leaving a 1/2-inch shell. Set aside the scooped out flesh in a bowl.
4. Place the zucchini flesh into a bowl and mash well. Mix in the tuna, onion, tomato, bread crumbs, egg, salt, and black pepper. Lightly stuff the zucchini shells with the tuna mixture. Drizzle about 1/2 teaspoon of olive oil over each stuffed zucchini half.
5. Bake in the preheated oven until the tops are slightly browned, 20 to 25 minutes.

WARM APPLE CINNAMON COBBLER

Servings: 6 | Prep: 20m | Cooks: 30m | Total: 50m

NUTRITION FACTS

Calories: 258 | Carbohydrates: 42.2g | Fat: 10.1g | Protein: 2.9g | Cholesterol: 0mg

INGREDIENTS

- 4 apples - peeled, cored and sliced
- 1 teaspoon baking powder
- 1 cup water
- 1/4 cup canola oil
- 2 teaspoons ground cinnamon
- 1 tablespoon honey

- 2 tablespoons cornstarch
- 1/2 cup lowfat buttermilk
- 1/4 cup fructose (fruit sugar)
- 1/2 cup lowfat buttermilk
- 1 cup whole wheat pastry flour

DIRECTIONS

1. Preheat oven to 375 degrees F (190 degrees C).
2. In a large saucepan over medium heat, combine the apples, water, cinnamon, cornstarch and fructose. Cook until apples are soft and mixture is thickened, about 10 minutes.
3. Pour the apple mixture into a casserole dish.
4. Prepare biscuit dough by combining the whole-wheat pastry flour and baking powder. Add the oil and stir until well mixed. Add the honey and buttermilk; stir with a fork until flour mixture is moist. Add additional milk if necessary.
5. Drop biscuit dough by tablespoons on top of apples. Bake for 20 minutes or until biscuits are golden brown. Serve warm.

BLACK-EYED PEAS SPICY STYLE

Servings: 3 | Prep: 10m | Cooks: 30m | Total: 40m

NUTRITION FACTS

Calories: 119 | Carbohydrates: 21.4g | Fat: 0.8g | Protein: 7.1g | Cholesterol: 0mg

INGREDIENTS

- 1 (15.5 ounce) can black-eyed peas with liquid
- minced jalapeno pepper to taste
- 1/2 onion, chopped
- ground black pepper to taste

DIRECTIONS

1. In a medium-size pot, combine black-eyed peas, onion, jalapeno peppers, and black pepper (to taste). Heat all ingredients to simmer, let cook 30 minutes. Enjoy!.

SPICY DILL POTATO SALAD

Servings: 12 | Prep: 30m | Cooks: 35m | Total: 3h35m

NUTRITION FACTS

Calories: 153 | Carbohydrates: 25.8g | Fat: 3.9g | Protein: 5.5g | Cholesterol: 63mg

INGREDIENTS

- 3 pounds russet potatoes, peeled and cubed
- 4 chipotle peppers in adobo sauce, chopped
- 4 eggs
- 1/4 cup adobo sauce from chipotle peppers
- 2 red bell peppers
- 8 sprigs fresh dill, chopped
- 2 green bell peppers
- 1 clove garlic, minced, or to taste
- 1 red onion
- 1 pinch ground cumin, or to taste
- 2 cups reduced-fat mayonnaise
- salt and ground black pepper to taste
- 1/2 cup horseradish mustard

DIRECTIONS

1. Place the potatoes into a large pot and cover with salted water. Bring to a boil over high heat, then reduce heat to medium-low, cover, and simmer until tender, 10 to 15 minutes. Drain and allow to steam dry for a minute or two. Place the potatoes into a large bowl, and chill in the refrigerator until cold, about 1 hour.
2. While the potatoes are boiling, place the eggs into a saucepan in a single layer and fill with water to cover the eggs by 1 inch. Cover the saucepan and bring the water to a boil over high heat. Once the water is boiling, remove from the heat and let the eggs stand in the hot water for 15 minutes. Pour out the hot water, then cool the eggs under cold running water in the sink. Peel once cold. Chop the eggs, and place into the bowl with the potatoes.
3. Preheat oven to 425 degrees F (220 degrees C). Cut the bell peppers in half, and remove the seeds, core, and stems. Place the bell peppers onto a baking sheet, cut sides down. Cut the onion in half, and place it onto the baking sheet, cut sides down.
4. Roast the peppers and onion in the preheated oven until the skin of the vegetables has charred in places, about 25 minutes. Remove any large pieces of burned skin, and chop the peppers and onions. Transfer into the bowl with the potatoes and eggs.
5. In a bowl, stir together the mayonnaise, horseradish mustard, chipotle peppers, adobo sauce, dill, garlic, cumin, and salt and pepper until thoroughly combined. Pour the dressing over the potato mixture, and lightly toss until the potatoes, eggs, and vegetables are thoroughly coated with dressing. Chill before serving.

BENGALI DHAL

Servings: 4 | Prep: 15m | Cooks: 30m | Total: 45m

NUTRITION FACTS

Calories: 224 | Carbohydrates: 34.3g | Fat: 4.1g | Protein: 13.2g | Cholesterol: 0mg

INGREDIENTS

- 1 cup red lentils
- 3/4 cup cherry tomatoes
- 3 cups water
- 1/2 teaspoon salt
- 1 cup onion, thinly sliced, divided
- 2 (2 inch) whole serrano chile peppers (optional)
- 4 cloves garlic, coarsely chopped, divided
- 1 tablespoon vegetable oil
- 1/2 teaspoon ground turmeric
- 2 tablespoons chopped cilantro
- 1 bay leaf

DIRECTIONS

1. Wash the lentils in a strainer. Combine the lentils and water in a saucepan over medium-high heat. Add half of the sliced onions and garlic, reserving the rest for later. Stir in the turmeric, bay leaf, tomatoes, and salt. Add the chiles, leaving them whole to add flavor or cut in half to add heat. When the mixture begins to boil, reduce the heat to a simmer. Cook until the lentils break apart and thicken slightly, about 20 minutes.
2. Meanwhile, in a skillet, heat the vegetable oil over medium heat until the oil shimmers. Add the reserved sliced onions; cook and stir until the onion has softened and turned translucent, about 5 minutes. Reduce heat to medium-low, and continue cooking and stirring until the onion is very tender and dark brown, 15 to 20 minutes more. Stir in the rest of the chopped garlic and cook, stirring constantly, until the garlic is fragrant and tender, about 2 minutes.
3. Pour the contents of the skillet into the cooked lentils and stir. Garnish with chopped cilantro.

FIESTA CHICKEN FROM UNCLE BEN'S®

Servings: 6 | Prep: 35m | Cooks: 35m | Total: 1h

NUTRITION FACTS

Calories: 94 | Carbohydrates: 16.1g | Fat: 2.8g | Protein: 3.2g | Cholesterol: 0mg

INGREDIENTS

- Nonstick cooking spray
- 3/4 cup red pepper, diced
- 3 cups water
- 1 cup chopped onion
- 1 1/2 tablespoons chili powder
- 3 cups UNCLE BEN'S® Fast & Natural™ Whole Grain Instant Brown Rice
- 1/4 cup chopped cilantro
- 6 chicken breast halves
- 3/4 cup salsa (mild)

- 1 cup corn kernels, frozen or canned

DIRECTIONS

1. Heat oil in a saute pan over medium heat. Add onion, and cook and stir for 3 minutes. Add tomatoes, zucchini, and green pepper. Stir. Season to taste with salt and black pepper. Reduce heat, cover, and simmer for 5 minutes.
2. Stir in rice and water. Cover, and cook over low heat for 20 minutes.

SUMMER FRUIT SALAD WITH A LEMON, HONEY, AND MINT DRESSING

Servings: 8 | Prep: 20m | Cooks: 1h | Total: 1h20m

NUTRITION FACTS

Calories: 99 | Carbohydrates: 24.8g | Fat: 0.5g | Protein: 1.5g | Cholesterol: 0mg

INGREDIENTS

- 4 cups cubed seeded watermelon
- 1 cup seedless grapes, halved
- 2 cups sliced fresh strawberries
- 2 lemons, juiced
- 2 large fresh peaches, cut into cubes
- 1/4 cup minced fresh mint (chocolate mint preferred)
- 2 large nectarines, cut into cubes
- 1/2 lemon, zested
- 1 red Anjou pear, cut into cubes
- 1 tablespoon honey (fireweed honey preferred)

DIRECTIONS

1. Combine watermelon, strawberries, peaches, nectarines, pear, and grapes in a large mixing bowl.
2. Whisk lemon juice, mint, lemon zest, and honey together in a small bowl; drizzle over the fruit mixture and toss to coat.
3. Refrigerate 1 hour before serving.

VANILLA GRANOLA

Servings: 16 | Prep: 10m | Cooks: 25m | Total: 35m

NUTRITION FACTS

Calories: 131 | Carbohydrates: 20g | Fat: 4.3g | Protein: 3.9g | Cholesterol: 0mg

INGREDIENTS

- non-stick cooking spray
- 1/4 teaspoon ground cinnamon
- 4 cups rolled oats
- 1 cup applesauce
- 1 cup sliced almonds
- 2 tablespoons white sugar
- 1/2 cup granular sucralose sweetener with brown sugar (such as Splenda® Brown Sugar Blend)
- 4 teaspoons vanilla extract
- 1/4 teaspoon salt

DIRECTIONS

1. Preheat oven to 300 degrees F (150 degrees C). Lightly spray large baking sheet with non-stick cooking spray.
2. Mix oats, almonds, sweetener, salt, and cinnamon in a large bowl.
3. Stir applesauce and sugar together in a small saucepan; bring to a simmer over medium heat and immediately remove from heat. Stir vanilla into the applesauce mixture; pour over the oats mixture and toss to coat. Spread the mixture onto the prepared baking dish.
4. Bake until golden brown, stirring occasionally, 20 to 30 minutes. Place baking sheet on a cooling rack until granola is completely cooled.

OVEN-FRIED BANANAS

Servings: 2 | Prep: 10m | Cooks: 10m | Total: 20m

NUTRITION FACTS

Calories: 119 | Carbohydrates: 25.6g | Fat: 1.4g | Protein: 2.6g | Cholesterol: 0mg

INGREDIENTS

- cooking spray
- 1/4 teaspoon ground ginger
- 1/4 cup dry bread crumbs
- 1 pinch salt
- 1 tablespoon granular no-calorie sucralose sweetener (such as Splenda®)
- 1 large banana, cut into slices
- 1/4 teaspoon ground cinnamon

DIRECTIONS

1. Preheat an oven to 425 degrees F (220 degrees C).
2. Line a baking sheet with parchment paper and spray with cooking spray.
3. Combine bread crumbs, no-calorie sweetener, cinnamon, ginger, and salt in a bowl.

4. Spray banana slices on both sides with the cooking spray.
5. Roll banana slices in the bread crumb mixture to coat, and arrange slices on the prepared baking sheet.
6. Lightly spray the banana slices again.
7. Bake in the preheated oven until crisp, 10 to 15 minutes.

SPICY BRUSSELS SPROUTS
Servings: 4 | Prep: 15m | Cooks: 30m | Total: 45m

NUTRITION FACTS

Calories: 64 | Carbohydrates: 13.4g | Fat: 0.4g | Protein: 4.1g | Cholesterol: 0mg

INGREDIENTS

- 1 pound Brussels sprouts
- 2 green onions, chopped
- 2 cloves garlic, thinly sliced
- 2 tablespoons Dijon mustard
- 1/2 teaspoon cayenne pepper
- 1 tablespoon lemon juice
- 1/2 teaspoon crushed red pepper flakes
- salt and ground black pepper to taste

DIRECTIONS

1. Place a steamer insert into a saucepan, and fill with water to just below the bottom of the steamer. Cover, and bring the water to a boil over high heat. Add the Brussels sprouts, and season with garlic, cayenne pepper, and red pepper flakes. Recover, and steam to your desired degree of tenderness, about 30 minutes for very tender.
2. Remove the Brussels sprouts from the steamer and place into a bowl. Add the green onions, mustard, and lemon juice. Season to taste with salt and pepper. Toss until evenly coated.

HONEY ORANGE GREEN BEANS
Servings: 4 | Prep: 15m | Cooks: 10m | Total: 45m

NUTRITION FACTS

Calories: 88 | Carbohydrates: 19.6g | Fat: 1.3g | Protein: 1.6g | Cholesterol: 0mg

INGREDIENTS

- 3 tablespoons honey

- 1 dash ground black pepper
- 1/2 orange, zested
- 1 tablespoon water
- 2 cloves garlic, minced
- 2 cups fresh green beans, trimmed
- 1 teaspoon soy sauce
- 1 teaspoon extra-virgin olive oil
- 1 1/2 teaspoons balsamic vinegar
- 1 tomato, diced

DIRECTIONS

1. Stir the honey, orange zest, garlic, soy sauce, balsamic vinegar, pepper, and water together in a bowl. Add the green beans and toss to coat. Allow to soak for 20 minutes, mixing every 5 minutes.
2. Heat the olive oil in a saucepan over low heat; add the green beans to the hot oil and cover the saucepan. Pour the green beans and sauce into the pan and cook, shaking the pan regularly, until the beans are slightly tender, about 5 minutes. Add the tomatoes to the green beans, replace the cover, and continue cooking until the green beans are cooked though yet slightly crispy, about 5 minutes more.

SPICY CHIPOTLE BLACK-EYED PEAS

Servings: 20 | Prep: 20m | Cooks: 8h | Total: 8h20m

NUTRITION FACTS

Calories: 156 | Carbohydrates: 26.9g | Fat: 2.7g | Protein: 9.2g | Cholesterol: 0mg

INGREDIENTS

- 2 tablespoons olive oil
- 2 (16 ounce) packages dry black-eyed peas
- 1 tablespoon balsamic vinegar
- 4 cups water
- 1 cup chopped orange bell pepper
- 4 teaspoons vegetable bouillon base (such as Better Than Bouillon® Vegetable Base)
- 1 cup chopped celery
- 1 (7 ounce) can chipotle peppers in adobo sauce, chopped, sauce reserved
- 1 cup chopped carrot
- 2 teaspoons liquid mesquite smoke flavoring
- 1 cup chopped onion
- 2 teaspoons ground cumin
- 1 teaspoon minced garlic
- 1/2 teaspoon ground black pepper

DIRECTIONS

1. Heat the olive oil and balsamic vinegar in a skillet; cook and stir the orange bell pepper, celery, carrot, onion, and garlic in the hot oil until the onion is translucent, 5 to 8 minutes. Transfer the mixture to a slow cooker; mix in the black-eyed peas, water, and vegetable base, stirring to dissolve the vegetable base. Stir in the chipotle peppers, about 1 tablespoon of the reserved adobo sauce (or to taste), liquid smoke, cumin, and black pepper.
2. Cook in the slow cooker on Low until the black-eyed peas are very tender and the flavors are blended, about 8 hours.

BEER SIMMERED BEANS

Servings: 6 | Prep: 10m | Cooks: 10m | Total: 20m

NUTRITION FACTS

Calories: 119 | Carbohydrates: 19.9g | Fat: 0.8g | Protein: 6.5g | Cholesterol: 0mg

INGREDIENTS

- 1 (15 ounce) can pinto beans, rinsed and drained
- 2 cloves garlic, minced
- 1 (15 ounce) can kidney beans, rinsed and drained
- 1 1/2 teaspoons cumin
- 1 cup light beer
- 1/4 teaspoon salt
- 2 jalapeno peppers, minced

DIRECTIONS

1. Combine pinto beans, kidney beans, beer, jalapenos, garlic, cumin, and salt in a large saucepan. Simmer for 10 minutes. Serve warm or chilled.

GRILLED CHICKEN CITRUS SALAD

Servings: 4 | Prep: 30m | Cooks: 15m | Total: 2h45m | Additional: 2h

NUTRITION FACTS

Calories: 238 | Carbohydrates: 26.1g | Fat: 2.2g | Protein: 30g | Cholesterol: 66mg

INGREDIENTS

- 1/2 cup orange juice
- 1 teaspoon white sugar
- 1/4 cup lime juice

- 4 (4 ounce) skinless, boneless chicken breast halves
- 2 shallots, minced
- 8 cups torn romaine lettuce
- 2 cloves garlic, minced
- 2 oranges - peeled, segmented, and chopped
- 1 teaspoon chili powder
- 2 stalks celery, sliced
- 1 teaspoon ground cumin
- 4 green onions, chopped

DIRECTIONS

1. In a mixing bowl, whisk together orange juice, lime juice, shallots, garlic, chili powder, cumin, and sugar. Pour 1/2 of this mixture into a large, resealable plastic bag, and add the chicken breasts. Seal, and refrigerate for at least 2 hours. Refrigerate the remaining dressing.
2. Preheat an outdoor grill for medium-high heat. In a large salad bowl, toss romaine lettuce with oranges, celery, and green onions. Set aside.
3. Lightly oil grate, and place chicken on grill. Discard the marinade from the chicken. Cook for 6 to 8 minutes each side, or until juices run clear when pierced with a fork. Remove chicken from grill, and slice into thin strips.
4. Toss salad with reserved dressing, and top with sliced chicken.

BOILED MUSTARD POTATOES

Servings: 6 | Prep: 15m | Cooks: 25m | Total: 40m

NUTRITION FACTS

Calories: 135 | Carbohydrates: 28.7g | Fat: 1g | Protein: 4.1g | Cholesterol: 0mg

INGREDIENTS

- 6 cups water
- 1/2 cup prepared yellow mustard, or to taste
- 1/2 teaspoon salt, or to taste
- 5 large Yukon Gold potatoes, peeled and halved

DIRECTIONS

1. Whisk the water, yellow mustard, and salt together in a large saucepan. Bring to a boil over medium heat, and stir in the potatoes. Reduce heat to medium-low, and simmer until tender, 25 to 30 minutes. Drain liquid, and serve.

A NEW GREEN BEAN CASSEROLE

Servings: 6 | Prep: 20m | Cooks: 1h | Total: 1h20m

NUTRITION FACTS

Calories: 97 | Carbohydrates: 19.5g | Fat: 1.3g | Protein: 4.6g | Cholesterol: 2mg

INGREDIENTS

- 1 1/2 pounds fresh green beans, trimmed
- 1 teaspoon dried basil
- 4 cups sliced onions
- 1 teaspoon dried oregano
- 2 tablespoons balsamic vinegar, or more if needed
- 1/4 cup shredded Parmesan cheese, or to taste
- 3 cloves garlic, chopped
- halved grape tomatoes
- 2 teaspoons white sugar

DIRECTIONS

1. Bring a large pot of lightly salted water to a boil; cook green beans at a boil until tender yet firm to the bite, 5 to 10 minutes; drain and transfer to a 9x13-inch dish.
2. Cook and stir onions, vinegar, garlic, sugar, basil, and oregano in a skillet over medium heat until onions are softened and translucent, about 5 minutes. Reduce heat to medium-low, and continue cooking and stirring until onions are very tender and dark brown, 15 to 20 minutes more.
3. Preheat oven to 400 degrees F (200 degrees C).
4. Spread onion mixture over green beans and top with Parmesan cheese. Arrange tomatoes, cut sides down, atop Parmesan cheese layer.
5. Bake in the preheated oven until cheese is melted and bubbling, about 35 minutes.

ZUCCHINI-TOMATO SAUTE

Servings: 1 | Prep: 5m | Cooks: 8h | Total: 8h5m

NUTRITION FACTS

Calories: 203 | Carbohydrates: 33.3g | Fat: 5g | Protein: 8.1g | Cholesterol: 0mg

INGREDIENTS

- 1/2 cup almond milk
- 2 tablespoons powdered peanut butter (such as PB2®)
- 1/4 cup fresh raspberries
- 1 1/2 teaspoons chia seeds
- 1/4 cup rolled oats
- 1 teaspoon white sugar

DIRECTIONS

1. Mix almond milk, raspberries, rolled oats, powdered peanut butter, chia seeds, and sugar together in a container. Cover and refrigerate until oats are soft, 8 hours to overnight.

CURRIED CREAM OF ANY VEGGIE SOUP

Servings: 6 | Prep: 15m | Cooks: 30m | Total: 45m

NUTRITION FACTS

Calories: 139 | Carbohydrates: 23.2g | Fat: 3.1g | Protein: 7g | Cholesterol: 2mg

INGREDIENTS

- 1 tablespoon vegetable oil
- 4 cups chopped mixed vegetables
- 1 onion, chopped
- 2 tablespoons all-purpose flour
- 1 clove garlic, minced
- 2 cups nonfat milk
- 1 tablespoon curry powder
- salt and pepper to taste
- 4 cups chicken broth

DIRECTIONS

1. Heat oil in a large saucepan over medium heat. Saute onion and garlic until tender. Stir in curry, and cook for 2 minutes, stirring constantly. Add broth and vegetables, and bring to a boil. Simmer 20 minutes, or until tender.
2. Dissolve flour in milk, then stir into the soup. Simmer until thickened. Season with salt and pepper.

COLORFUL BULGUR SALAD

Servings: 4 | Prep: 15m | Cooks: 10m | Total: 3h20m

NUTRITION FACTS

Calories: 65 | Carbohydrates: 13.8g | Fat: 0.7g | Protein: 2.9g | Cholesterol: 0mg

INGREDIENTS

- 1/2 cup cracked bulgur wheat
- 3 green onions, thinly sliced
- 1/2 cup chicken broth
- 3 tablespoons fresh lime juice
- 1 small cucumber, seeded and chopped
- 3/4 tablespoon chili powder

- 1 tomato, chopped
- 1 pinch garlic powder
- 1 carrot, shredded

DIRECTIONS

1. Place bulgur in a colander and rinse under cold running water. Drain and transfer to a small bowl.
2. In a small saucepan bring the chicken broth to a boil. Stir in the bulgur, remove from the heat and let stand for 1 hour.
3. Stir in the cucumbers, tomatoes, carrots, and green onions into the bulgur.
4. In a small bowl whisk the lime juice, chili powder and garlic powder together. Pour over the bulgur mixture and stir until combined. Cover and chill for 2 hours before serving. Stir before serving.

REDUCED FAT FRENCH TOAST

Servings: 6 | Prep: 5m | Cooks: 10m | Total: 15m

NUTRITION FACTS

Calories: 77 | Carbohydrates: 11.9g | Fat: 1.3g | Protein: 5.4g | Cholesterol: <1mg

INGREDIENTS

- 1/2 cup egg substitute
- 1/2 teaspoon ground cinnamon
- 2/3 cup skim milk
- 6 slices reduced calorie white bread
- 1 teaspoon vanilla extract

DIRECTIONS

1. Beat together egg substitute, milk, vanilla and cinnamon. Dip bread slices in egg mixture until both sides are soaked.
2. Spray a skillet or frying pan with cooking spray and heat over medium high heat. Place bread slices into pan and cook until golden brown on both sides .

OVEN BAKED VEGETABLES

Servings: 6 | Prep: 10m | Cooks: 25m | Total: 35m

NUTRITION FACTS

Calories: 98 | Carbohydrates: 22.5g | Fat: 0.2g | Protein: 2.1g | Cholesterol: 0mg

INGREDIENTS

- 1 vegetable cooking spray

- 1/3 cup fat free Italian-style dressing
- 2 potatoes, cubed
- 1/8 teaspoon garlic salt
- 1 carrot, sliced
- 1/4 teaspoon cayenne pepper
- 2 onions, sliced
- 1/8 teaspoon onion salt
- 1 green bell pepper, chopped

DIRECTIONS

1. Preheat oven to 350 degrees F (175 degrees C). Spray a 9 x 13 inch baking pan with cooking spray.
2. In prepared pan combine potatoes, carrots, onions and bell pepper.
3. In a small bowl combine Italian dressing, garlic salt, cayenne pepper and onion salt. Pour over vegetables.
4. Bake, covered, for 15 minutes. Uncover, stir and bake for 10 minutes more.

CARIBBEAN SLAW

Servings: 8 | Prep: 20m | Cooks: 1h | Total: 1h20m

NUTRITION FACTS

Calories: 61 | Carbohydrates: 13.1g | Fat: 0.6g | Protein: 2.1g | Cholesterol: <1mg

INGREDIENTS

- 1/2 head green cabbage, shredded
- 2 tablespoons reduced-fat mayonnaise
- 1 red bell pepper, thinly sliced
- 1 tablespoon prepared yellow mustard
- 1/2 red onion, thinly sliced
- 1 tablespoon apple cider vinegar
- 2 carrots, peeled and shredded
- 1 teaspoon agave nectar
- 1 mango - peeled, seeded, and diced
- salt and black pepper to taste
- 1/2 cup fresh cilantro, chopped
- 1 dash habanero hot sauce, or more to taste
- 1/3 cup nonfat plain yogurt

DIRECTIONS

1. Toss the cabbage, red bell pepper, red onion, carrots, mango, and cilantro together in a large bowl.

2. Whisk the yogurt, mayonnaise, mustard, cider vinegar, agave nectar, salt, pepper, and hot sauce together in a small bowl; pour over the cabbage mixture and toss to coat. Allow the slaw to marinate in the refrigerator for at least 1 hour to allow the flavors to combine.

AIR FRYER GARLIC AND PARSLEY BABY POTATOES
Servings: 5 | Prep: 5m | Cooks: 20m | Total: 25m

NUTRITION FACTS

Calories: 89 | Carbohydrates: 20.1g | Fat: 0.1g | Protein: 2.4g | Cholesterol: 0mg

INGREDIENTS

- 1 pound baby potatoes, cut into quarters
- 1/2 teaspoon granulated garlic
- 1 tablespoon avocado oil
- 1/2 teaspoon dried parsley
- 1/4 teaspoon salt

DIRECTIONS

1. Preheat an air fryer to 350 degrees F (175 degrees C).
2. Combine potatoes and oil in a bowl and toss to coat. Add 1/4 teaspoon granulated garlic and 1/4 teaspoon parsley and toss to coat. Repeat with remaining garlic and parsley. Pour potatoes into the air fryer basket.
3. Place the basket in the air fryer and cook, tossing occasionally, until golden brown, about 20 to 25 minutes.

APPLE AND PUMPKIN DESSERT
Servings: 1 | Prep: 5m | Cooks: 4m | Total: 9m

NUTRITION FACTS

Calories: 88 | Carbohydrates: 23.8g | Fat: 0.4g | Protein: 1.2g | Cholesterol: 0mg

INGREDIENTS

- 2 (1 gram) packets sugar substitute
- 1/4 cup canned pumpkin
- 1 teaspoon pumpkin pie spice
- 2 tablespoons water
- 1 Granny Smith apple - peeled, cored and chopped

DIRECTIONS

1. Sprinkle 1/3 packet of sugar substitute and 1/3 teaspoon pumpkin pie spice in the bottom of a microwave-safe bowl. Layer 1/4 of the apple pieces into the bowl; repeat. Spread the pumpkin over the apples. Sprinkle the remaining sugar substitute and pumpkin pie spice on the pumpkin. Top with the remaining apples. Pour the water over the mixture.
2. Cook in microwave on high for 3 1/2 minutes, stirring every minute.

FRUITY TUNA SALAD
Servings: 6 | Prep: 10m | Cooks: 1h | Total: 1h10m

NUTRITION FACTS

Calories: 159 | Carbohydrates: 27.2g | Fat: 0.8g | Protein: 12.6g | Cholesterol: 14mg

INGREDIENTS

- 2 (5 ounce) cans tuna, drained
- 1/2 cup lemon yogurt
- 1 cup chopped dates
- 1 tablespoon minced onion
- 1 1/2 cups chopped celery
- 2 teaspoons lemon juice
- 1 large apple - peeled, cored and diced
- 1 teaspoon ground curry powder

DIRECTIONS

1. In a large bowl, mix the tuna, dates, celery and apple.
2. In a separate bowl, whisk together the yogurt, onion, lemon juice, and curry powder. Pour over tuna mixture and gently toss to coat. Refrigerate 1 hour, or until chilled.

INSTANT POT® APPLE PIE STEEL CUT OATS
Servings: 4 | Prep: 5m | Cooks: 15m | Total: 30m

NUTRITION FACTS

Calories: 171 | Carbohydrates: 32.6g | Fat: 2.6g | Protein: 5.1g | Cholesterol: 0mg

INGREDIENTS

- 3 cups water
- 1 1/2 teaspoons ground cinnamon
- 1 cup steel-cut oats
- 1/2 teaspoon salt
- 1 apple, or more to taste, chopped

- 1/4 teaspoon ground nutmeg

DIRECTIONS

1. Combine water, oats, apple, cinnamon, salt, and nutmeg in a multi-functional pressure cooker (such as Instant Pot(R)). Close and lock the lid. Seal vent. Select Manual function; set timer for 5 minutes. Allow 10 to 15 minutes for pressure to build.
2. Release pressure using the natural-release method according to manufacturer's instructions, about 10 minutes. Release remaining pressure naturally. Stir and remove pot carefully with oven mitts.

EASY SOUTHERN FRIED GREEN TOMATOES
Servings: 8 | Prep: 15m | Cooks: 10m | Total: 25m

NUTRITION FACTS

Calories: 189 | Carbohydrates: 31.5g | Fat: 4.7g | Protein: 5.8g | Cholesterol: 46mg

INGREDIENTS

- waxed paper
- sea salt to taste
- 2 large eggs
- freshly ground black pepper to taste
- 2 tablespoons water
- 2 pounds green tomatoes, sliced
- 1 cup all-purpose flour
- 1 cup canola oil for frying, or as needed
- 1 cup yellow cornmeal

DIRECTIONS

1. Line a baking sheet with waxed paper.
2. Beat eggs and water in a shallow bowl. Place flour and cornmeal in 2 separate shallow bowls. Season cornmeal with salt and pepper.
3. Dip each tomato slice into flour, then dip into egg mixture. Press tomato into cornmeal mixture, shaking off excess. Transfer tomato to prepared baking sheet. Repeat with remaining tomato slices, arranging tomatoes in a single layer.
4. Heat about 1/4 inch canola oil in a large skillet over medium heat until oil begins to shimmer. Fry tomatoes in batches until golden and crisp, 3 to 4 minutes per side. Drain on paper towel-lined plates. Repeat with remaining tomatoes.

PROTEIN-PACKED SPICY VEGAN QUINOA WITH EDAMAME
Servings: 8 | Prep: 15m | Cooks: 30m | Total: 45m

NUTRITION FACTS

Calories: 94 | Carbohydrates: 16.1g | Fat: 2.8g | Protein: 3.2g | Cholesterol: 0mg

INGREDIENTS

- 3 1/2 cups water
- 2 bell peppers, chopped
- 2 cups quinoa, rinsed
- 2 tablespoons minced fresh ginger
- 4 teaspoons vegetable bouillon (such as Better Than Bouillon®)
- 6 cloves garlic, minced
- 2 1/2 cups frozen shelled edamame (green soybeans)
- 1/4 cup reduced-sodium soy sauce
- 1 tablespoon olive oil
- 2 tablespoons chopped fresh cilantro
- 2 sweet onions, chopped
- 1 tablespoon hot chile paste (such as sambal oelek), or to taste (optional)

DIRECTIONS

1. Bring water, quinoa, and vegetable bouillon to a boil in a large pot; stir in edamame, cover, and simmer until quinoa is tender, 15 to 20 minutes.
2. Heat olive oil in a large skillet over medium heat; cook and stir onions and bell peppers until onions are translucent, about 5 minutes. Add ginger and garlic; cook and stir until fragrant, about 2 minutes. Remove from heat; stir in soy sauce, cilantro, and chile paste.
3. Stir onion mixture into quinoa mixture; simmer, stirring occasionally, until excess broth has been absorbed, about 5 minutes.

PROTEIN-PACKED SPICY VEGAN QUINOA WITH EDAMAME

Servings: 8 | Prep: 15m | Cooks: 30m | Total: 45m

NUTRITION FACTS

Calories: 206 | Carbohydrates: 34.9g | Fat: 4.6g | Protein: 7.3g | Cholesterol: 0mg

INGREDIENTS

- 3 1/2 cups water
- 2 bell peppers, chopped
- 2 cups quinoa, rinsed
- 2 tablespoons minced fresh ginger

- 4 teaspoons vegetable bouillon (such as Better Than Bouillon®)
- 6 cloves garlic, minced
- 2 1/2 cups frozen shelled edamame (green soybeans)
- 1/4 cup reduced-sodium soy sauce
- 1 tablespoon olive oil
- 2 tablespoons chopped fresh cilantro
- 2 sweet onions, chopped
- 1 tablespoon hot chile paste (such as sambal oelek), or to taste (optional)

DIRECTIONS

1. Bring water, quinoa, and vegetable bouillon to a boil in a large pot; stir in edamame, cover, and simmer until quinoa is tender, 15 to 20 minutes.
2. Heat olive oil in a large skillet over medium heat; cook and stir onions and bell peppers until onions are translucent, about 5 minutes. Add ginger and garlic; cook and stir until fragrant, about 2 minutes. Remove from heat; stir in soy sauce, cilantro, and chile paste.
3. Stir onion mixture into quinoa mixture; simmer, stirring occasionally, until excess broth has been absorbed, about 5 minutes.

CALICO SLAW

Servings: 8 | Prep: 20m | Cooks: 30m | Total: 50m

NUTRITION FACTS

Calories: 81 | Carbohydrates: 19.4g | Fat: 0.3g | Protein: 2.2g | Cholesterol: 0mg

INGREDIENTS

- 1 medium head green cabbage, shredded
- 1 Golden Delicious apple, cored and chopped
- 3 carrots, shredded
- 2 tablespoons apple cider vinegar
- 1 green bell pepper, seeded and thinly sliced
- 2 tablespoons white sugar
- 1 red bell pepper, seeded and thinly sliced
- 1/2 teaspoon fine sea salt
- 1 yellow bell pepper, seeded and thinly sliced
- ground black pepper, to taste
- 1 Red Delicious apple, cored and chopped

DIRECTIONS

1. Toss the cabbage, carrots, green bell pepper, red bell pepper, Red Delicious apple, and Golden Delicious apple together in a large bowl.

2. Whisk the apple cider vinegar, sugar, and sea salt together in a small bowl; season with black pepper. Pour the vinegar mixture over the cabbage mixture and gently toss to coat. Cover the bowl with plastic wrap and refrigerate at least 30 minutes.

BANANA CHIA PUDDING
Servings: 6 | Prep: 10m | Cooks: 2h | Total: 2h10m

NUTRITION FACTS

Calories: 112 | Carbohydrates: 20.5g | Fat: 3.4g | Protein: 1.6g | Cholesterol: 0mg

INGREDIENTS

- 1 1/2 cups vanilla-flavored flax milk
- 3 tablespoons honey
- 1 large banana, cut in chunks
- 1 teaspoon vanilla extract
- 7 tablespoons chia seeds
- 1/8 teaspoon sea salt

DIRECTIONS

1. Put milk, banana, chia seeds, honey, vanilla extract, and sea salt in respective order in the blender; blend until smooth. Pour mixture into a bowl and refrigerate until thickened, at least 2 hours. Spoon mixture into small bowls to serve.

DUCK FAT-ROASTED BRUSSELS SPROUTS
Servings: 4 | Prep: 20m | Cooks: 15m | Total: 35m

NUTRITION FACTS

Calories: 125 | Carbohydrates: 23.4g | Fat: 3.1g | Protein: 8g | Cholesterol: 2mg

INGREDIENTS

- 2 tablespoons duck fat, or more as needed
- 1 pinch cayenne pepper, or more to taste
- 2 pounds Brussels sprouts, trimmed and halved lengthwise
- 1 lemon, juiced
- salt and freshly ground black pepper to taste

DIRECTIONS

1. Preheat an oven to 450 degrees F (230 degrees C). Line a baking sheet with parchment paper or a silicone baking mat.

2. Heat duck fat in a small saucepan until melted.
3. Combine Brussels sprouts, salt, black pepper, cayenne pepper, and melted duck fat in a large bowl until Brussels sprouts are evenly coated. Transfer to the prepared baking sheet.
4. Bake in the preheated oven until Brussels sprouts are browned and tender, but still slightly firm, 15 to 20 minutes. Flip Brussels sprouts over halfway through. Top with freshly squeezed lemon juice.

INSTANT POT® STEAMED ARTICHOKES
Servings: 4 | Prep: 5m | Cooks: 20m | Total: 30m

NUTRITION FACTS

Calories: 64 | Carbohydrates: 14.6g | Fat: 0.2g | Protein: 4.3g | Cholesterol: 0mg

INGREDIENTS

- 1 cup water
- 1/2 teaspoon salt
- 2 cloves garlic
- 4 artichokes, trimmed and stemmed
- 1 bay leaf
- 2 tablespoons lemon juice

DIRECTIONS

1. Combine water, garlic, bay leaf, and salt inside a multi-functional pressure cooker (such as Instant Pot(R)). Place steamer in the pot. Add artichokes, trimmed top facing up; drizzle with lemon juice. Close and lock the lid. Select high pressure according to manufacturer's instructions; set timer for 10 minutes. Allow 10 to 15 minutes for pressure to build.
2. Release pressure carefully using the quick-release method according to manufacturer's instructions, about 5 minutes. Unlock and remove lid.
3. Cool until easily handled. Pull off outer petals one at a time. Pull through teeth to remove the soft portion of the petal. Discard remaining petal. Spoon out fuzzy center near the stem and discard. Eat the bottom whole or cut into pieces.

VEGGIE-PACKED MEATLOAF WITH QUINOA
Servings: 8 | Prep: 20m | Cooks: 55m | Total: 1h20m

NUTRITION FACTS

Calories: 232 | Carbohydrates: 22.9g | Fat: 2.8g | Protein: 27.8g | Cholesterol: 82mg

INGREDIENTS

- 1 onion, quartered
- 1 1/2 pounds lean ground meat (turkey or chicken)

- 4 cloves garlic, peeled
- 1 1/4 cups quinoa, cooked then cooled
- 1 large carrot, quartered
- 3 tablespoons low-sodium soy sauce
- 1 celery stalk, quartered
- 1/2 teaspoon ground black pepper
- 2 1/2 cups baby spinach
- 1/4 cup ketchup or barbecue sauce
- 1 egg, lightly beaten

DIRECTIONS

1. Preheat the oven to 425 degrees F and line a small baking sheet with parchment paper.
2. Place onion and garlic in a food processor and pulse until finely chopped. Transfer to a large skillet. Add carrot and celery to the food processor, and pulse until chopped. Add spinach and pulse a few times more. Add to the skillet. Place the skillet over medium heat and cook, stirring until vegetables release liquid. Continue cooking until liquid evaporates and vegetables begin to brown, about 8 minutes; add water a tablespoon at a time, if necessary, to keep vegetables from sticking. Transfer to a large bowl.
3. Add egg, ground meat, quinoa, soy sauce and black pepper to the bowl, and mix gently with your hands. Scrape mixture onto the baking sheet and form into a loaf approximately 4 inches wide and 10 inches long; wet your hands if the mixture is very sticky. Spread top of loaf with ketchup or barbecue sauce. Bake until cooked through and browned, about 40 minutes. Cool 5 minutes before slicing.

BONE BROTH

Servings: 8 | Prep: 10m | Cooks: 1d30m | Total: 1d40m

NUTRITION FACTS

Calories: 49 | Carbohydrates: 11.4g | Fat: 0.2g | Protein: 1.8g | Cholesterol: 0mg

INGREDIENTS

- cooking spray
- 2 onions, thickly sliced
- 1 (6 ounce) can tomato paste
- 2 carrots
- 2 pounds beef bones
- 3 cloves garlic, crushed
- 6 cups cool water, or as needed
- 2 bay leaves

DIRECTIONS

1. Preheat oven to 400 degrees F (200 degrees C). Spray a roasting pan with cooking spray.
2. Spread tomato paste onto beef bones and place in the prepared roasting pan.
3. Bake in the preheated oven until bones begin to brown, about 30 minutes.
4. Transfer bones to a slow cooker and pour in enough water to cover bones. Add onions, carrots, garlic, and bay leaves to broth mixture.
5. Cook on Low for at least 24 hours.
6. Strain broth through a fine-mesh strainer into a container and refrigerate.

"SKINNY" CHICKEN TACOS
Servings: 4 | Prep: 15m | Cooks: 10m | Total: 35m | Additional: 10m

NUTRITION FACTS

Calories: 272 | Carbohydrates: 37.2g | Fat: 3.9g | Protein: 29.3g | Cholesterol: 65mg

INGREDIENTS

- 1 pound thinly sliced chicken breasts, cut into thin strips
- 2 red bell peppers, cut into thin strips
- 3 limes, juiced, divided
- 1 red onion, thinly sliced
- 2 teaspoons ground cumin, divided
- 2 jalapeno peppers - stemmed, seeded, and thinly sliced
- 2 teaspoons garlic powder, divided
- 4 multi-grain tortillas, or more to taste
- 2 teaspoons ground chipotle pepper, divided
- 1 bunch cilantro, chopped

DIRECTIONS

1. Combine chicken, juice of 1 lime, 1 teaspoon cumin, 1 teaspoon garlic powder, and 1 teaspoon chipotle pepper in a bowl; allow to marinate for 10 minutes.
2. Saute red bell peppers, onion, jalapeno peppers, juice of 1 lime, 1 teaspoon cumin, 1 teaspoon garlic powder, and 1 teaspoon chipotle pepper in a large non-stick skillet over medium-high heat until vegetables are tender yet crisp, about 5 minutes.
3. Transfer chicken mixture to a separate non-stick skillet over medium-high heat; saute until chicken is no longer pink in the center, 5 to 10 minutes.
4. Layer tortillas between paper towels on a microwave-safe plate; heat in microwave until warmed, 10 to 20 seconds.
5. Spoon vegetables and chicken onto tortillas; top with cilantro and lime juice.

TANGY JICAMA SLAW
Servings: 6 | Prep: 15m | Cooks: 10m | Total: 25m

NUTRITION FACTS

Calories: 67 | Carbohydrates: 16.6g | Fat: 0.2g | Protein: 1.3g | Cholesterol: 0mg

INGREDIENTS

- 1 jicama, peeled and chopped
- 1 lemon, juiced
- 1/4 cup fresh cilantro leaves, minced
- 1 (11 ounce) can mandarin orange segments, drained, liquid reserved
- 1 large lime, juiced
- salt to taste

DIRECTIONS

1. Combine the jicama, cilantro, lime juice, lemon juice, and mandarin orange segments with a small amount of the syrup from the can in a bowl; mix to evenly coat. Allow mixture to sit 10 minutes. Season with salt and stir just before serving.

KIWI SALSA

Servings: 6 | Prep: 15m | Cooks: 1h | Total: 1h15m

NUTRITION FACTS

Calories: 78 | Carbohydrates: 14g | Fat: 2.7g | Protein: 1.1g | Cholesterol: 0mg

INGREDIENTS

- 6 kiwis, peeled and diced
- 1 tablespoon olive oil
- 1 small onion, diced
- 1 teaspoon honey
- 1 jalapeno pepper, diced
- 1/2 teaspoon cumin
- 2 tablespoons lime juice
- 1/2 teaspoon curry powder

DIRECTIONS

1. Mix kiwi, onion, jalapeno pepper, lime juice, olive oil, honey, cumin, and curry powder together in bowl. Cover and allow to rest for 1 hour at room temperature. Refrigerate until ready to serve.

POLLO CON NOPALES (CHICKEN AND CACTUS)

Servings: 2 | Prep: 10m | Cooks: 20m | Total: 30m

NUTRITION FACTS

Calories: 174 | Carbohydrates: 11.9g | Fat: 3.2g | Protein: 25.7g | Cholesterol: 59mg

INGREDIENTS

- 2 skinless, boneless chicken breast halves
- 3 fresh jalapeno peppers, seeded
- 3 fresh tomatillos, husks removed
- 1 (16 ounce) jar canned nopales (cactus), drained

DIRECTIONS

1. Fill a pot with water and bring to a boil. Cook the chicken breasts in the boiling water until no longer pink in the center and the juices run clear, about 10 minutes. An instant-read thermometer inserted into the center should read at least 165 degrees F (74 degrees C). Drain and set aside to cool. Once cool, shred the chicken into small strands.
2. Fill the pot again with water and bring to a boil. Cook the tomatillos, jalapeno peppers, and nopales in the boiling water until the vegetables are all tender, about 5 minutes. Drain.
3. Blend the tomatillos and jalapeno peppers in a blender until smooth; pour into the pot with the shredded chicken and place over medium heat. Cut the nopales into small dice and add to the mixture. Allow the mixture to simmer until completely reheated, about 5 minutes.

MEXICAN MANGO

Servings: 2 | Prep: 5m | Cooks: 10m | Total: 15m

NUTRITION FACTS

Calories: 85 | Carbohydrates: 21.7g | Fat: 0.9g | Protein: 1.1g | Cholesterol: 0mg

INGREDIENTS

- 1/4 cup water
- 3 tablespoons lemon juice
- 1 tablespoon chili powder
- 1 mango - peeled, seeded, and sliced
- 1 pinch salt

DIRECTIONS

1. Bring water to a boil in a small saucepan. Stir in chili powder, salt, and lemon juice until smooth and hot. Add sliced mango and toss to coat; allow to soak up the chili sauce for a few minutes before serving.

Printed in the USA
CPSIA information can be obtained
at www.ICGtesting.com
LVHW081009280324
775738LV00010B/395

9 798513 721444